WOMEN LOOK AT PSYCHIATRY

edited by
Dorothy E. Smith
& Sara J. David

editorial assistance from
Barbara Joyce
Julia Meadows
Debbie Nilson
Eve-Lynne Rubin

Press Gang Publishers

Women Look at Psychiatry ISBN 0 88974 000 3 pb.
ISBN 0 88974 001 1 cl.

First printing March 1976
Second printing August 1977

Cover design by Pat Smith
Drawings by Lindy Filkow
Layout by the Vancouver Women's Publishing Project
Typeset by Anno Delaney of Makara Publishing and Design Co-operative
Printed and published in Canada by the Press Gang collective (Sarah Davidson, Ina Dennekamp, Barbara Farkas, Jane MacDermot, Lou Nelson, Pat Smith)

Some financial assistance provided by the Department of Manpower and Immigration through the OFY Programme, and the Vancouver Mental Patients' Association

All royalties go to the B.C. Women's Studies Research Association

TABLE OF CONTENTS

INTRODUCTION

This book is made up of articles written by women who are or have been involved with psychiatry, either professionally or as patients or both. It is a critical book, concerned with how psychiatry has contributed to women's oppression and with ways of changing that. Its aim is to make visible how current psychiatric practice affects women, and to offer readers a chance to learn from women's experiences in doing it differently. We want to offer women concepts, ideas, examples, critiques, information, understandings which they can use for thinking, talking with others, arguing, and criticizing. The idea of this book came partly from the experience of women in the Vancouver area who had tried to find ways of expressing what they knew intuitively, of being heard at psychiatric conferences, and of organizing sources of help for women. They felt that women did not have and needed means of analysis, information, models of how to proceed and that they also wanted a book to which they could refer other women.

In a sense the book started in 1973 when Meredith Kimball and Dorothy Smith talked at the first session of a series of public lectures on Madness in Society, organized by Hank Rosenthal for the University of British Columbia Continuing Education Dept. Rita MacDonald attended that session. She taped it and listened to the tapes many times. She wanted to be able to incorporate into her practice the kind of political analysis which Meredith and Dorothy had made. Seeing that women needed ideas to think about and analyze the world from the perspective of their experience and interests and to develop their practice came for Dorothy Smith partly out of talking with Rita about her work. The session summarized in "A Feminist Therapy Session" is an instance of the kind of work Rita began to do in working this out. It is an instance also of one way in which the book is intended to be used.

When we first tried to put it together, we discovered that what we had was uniformly critical and negative. There was very little to offer which showed the way toward alternative and feminist approaches to psychotherapy. Over the two years that the pieces of the book sat around in various people's files and heads, this has changed radically. As you'll see, there are now not only women doing therapy who have things to say about how to go about feminist therapy but also at least one instance of a woman who has experienced both the old and the new and can tell us about the difference for her. For this reason, we have chosen to end the book with Barbara Joyce's, "I'm Not Crazy After All."

This anthology includes both personal accounts by women of in-patient and out-patient psychiatric treatment and analyses of such intervention. It begins by criticizing the destructiveness of traditional approaches to women seeking psychiatric help and goes on to suggest alternate non-sexist models of treatment.

The anthology is intended to present a feminist analysis of the psychiatric oppression of women. While the personal accounts selected do not always explicitly differentiate poor therapy from sexist therapy, they were selected for inclusion because they tell about psychiatry as women experience it.

Women who have received psychiatric treatment can, we hope, find in this book confirmation of their intuitions about their own psychiatric experiences; women seeking treatment may find here both an analysis of what may be in store and a basis for assessing the alternatives; women in general may be able to discover some further aspects of the forces which oppress them in capitalist society and increase their awareness of what other women have been working on to break out of these. We hope also that this will be used by therapists who are seeking non-sexist means of therapy and finally that it might be a source for both therapists and their patients of criticism of those ways of doing psychiatry which need change.

Some of the articles disagree with one another and some are factually contradictory. We have not tried to impose editorial consistency. The papers were written at different times and even over this short period of two years women have been very active in developing this whole area of their understanding of our situation. This book brings together the work of women in western Canada. We have wanted them to speak for themselves and to represent rather than gloss over their disagreements with each other or ours with them.

Dorothy E. Smith and Sara David

WOMEN & PSYCHIATRY

Dorothy E. Smith

The relation "women and psychiatry" cannot be understood in isolation from the larger social organization of North American society. The consequences and implications of psychiatry are not restricted to what is recognized in ideology or in the routine practices of hospital, clinic and office as its professional jurisdiction. They depend also upon the lived contexts in which the patient experiences that relation. Psychiatric ideologies and practices work within and constitute a specialized domain, but in the lives of its practitioners and of those it "treats", psychiatry takes on its determinate character as part of a larger social organization bringing it into unseen relations with other aspects of the human condition. What psychiatry actually does do is a product not of its professionally defined intentions alone, but also of the socially determinate contexts in which they are received and lived by patients and others over whom its influences extend. What it means and how it has consequences cannot be read simply from its own texts, nor understood in the terms of its own discourse, what it claims to do and how it plans, systematizes and justifies its practices.

Women and men in western industrialized society are situated differently and encounter the world from different bases of experience. The division between them is drawn along biological lines but it is not biologically determined. This of course is true of all societies. But there are special features to the division in our society. First – the images, vocabularies, conceptual practices, symbols, knowledges and methods of knowing the world do not arise directly out of and in relation to the everyday world of experience. They are produced as a specialized enterprise by various forms of corporate or professional organization. Specially qualified or talented men produce these images, vocabularies, concepts, symbols, knowledges, etcetera, for others to use, to know, to think and image with. Second – the modes in which western industrialized societies are ruled, governed, managed and administered are also symbolic. Men act in words or other symbolic forms to get things done, some of which begin and end in words or other symbolic forms. This practice of ruling requires, in addition, the production of a reality which will correspond and answer to its practice. It requires a world which can be known in that symbolic mode of action as information, facts, news, data and the like. What is or can be recognized in this mode has authoritative recognition. It assumes a special status. It has been accorded the "accent of reality" and becomes 'objective.'

Psychiatry and psychiatric institutions play a special part in this way of ordering and controlling events and people. They do so both by treating people and by helping to create the ideological terms in which human realities may be made known in forms corresponding to its practices of control. These ideologies appear in a variety of forms, and at a variety of levels of sophistication. They appear in the professional journals, in the popular and semi-popular literature of paperback books, women's magazines and columns such as that of Ann Landers.

This practice of ruling is largely if not exclusively the prerogative of men. As a world, it is occupied, practiced, thought and performed almost exclusively by men. Men appropriate these symbolic forms of action and they appropriate the work of producing the ideological forms in which what gets done is known and thought of. Our means of knowing and speaking of ourselves and our world are written for us by men who occupy a special place in it. They view the world and the others who are part of its making from this position in it. They have the authority to produce that view as an objective account of reality.[1]

For a given class of men, producing ideological forms for others to use and practicing the symbolic modes of getting things done are their everyday world of working. These are a fundamental aspect of their experience. They are located in that mode. Their perspective upon the world is shaped by their special position in it. They look out on a world the character and distinctive features of which are given already by this organization.

The history and contemporary experience of women is not fully voiced because the position of women is marginal and subservient to this male-appropriated practice of ruling. Women have been unable to develop means of expression out of their own activities and experience because they have been deprived of the means to do so. The ideologies available to them for thinking about their experience and the world as it

 becomes for them have been made up for them and largely

from outside. The perspective implicit in these ideologies views women from outside themselves and in a subservient relation to the enterprises of men.

Women's novels, women's magazines, the women's section of the newspapers, the representations of women in advertising, in movies, in children's stories, as well as in the social sciences, take for granted a role for women which is complementary to and derived from their relation to men. De Beauvoir has given us terms which make this observable. She tells us that women learn to know and practice themselves only as Other vis-à-vis men as Subject. They have not developed an authentic basis originating with themselves. In knowing themselves only in relation to men and only in forms produced for them by men, they are alienated from themselves and their experience.[2]

The movie *Souffle au Coeur* demonstrates in an unusually comprehensive form the array of roles in which women are defined relative to the enterprise and interests of men. The story, a comedy, turns on an incestuous relation between a young and very beautiful mother and her teenage son. Women's roles in the movies are displayed as if they made up the totality of women's existence. We are not shown even the possibility of an autonomous basis for their existence.

Here is the array: first, there is the ambiguous role of mother passing over into that of mistress; mother also plays the role of mistress vis-à-vis a nebulous lover; there is the role of secretary to husband and father which passes over into that of mistress to the boss; there is the role of whore which has the merit of simplicity since she plays whore and nothing else; there is the role of servant which is likewise simple; and finally since father/husband is a gynecologist, there is the role of patient. All these ways of being a woman are defined here solely as they are relevant to the interests, needs and enterprises of men. Women exist in *Souffle au Coeur* only in relation to men. Even the incestuous passage between mother and son serves only to release him into a wider sexual activity and into the adult world in which men use women, and women's existence is defined by their uses to men.

The women in this paradigmatic movie have no centre in relation to which men might appear as complements to *their* enterprise. Men stand at a centre from which women are surveyed and given determinate being. Women do not look back at men from a place of their own.[3] This is a model, for middle class women in particular, of how they are related to men and to the world of men. They have learned to subordinate their understanding of themselves and their experience to a conception of who they are that comes from outside. It is one that gives them no alternative to seeing themselves from outside and in terms of their uses to others.

How then may women understand their situation? What vocabularies and concepts are available to them to think about their world and to speak from their experience? Where are the expressive forms and the images and symbols which are capable of realizing the special character of their experience? How can they formulate their lives and feelings so that they can speak to one another of what they have in common, declare who they are, make claims, speak with authority of their condition and recognize themselves fully in what is said? The relation "women and psychiatry" must be understood in the context of the radical deprivation women have suffered of the means to speak of themselves and their condition.

II

Sociologists view psychiatry as among the "mechanisms of social control" in contemporary society. It specializes in problems of control arising when individuals act in ways which don't fit with the institutionalized order. It deals with the leakages at the edges of the publically conceived and sanctioned order, with gaps in the jurisdictions of other "mechanisms" of control and with problems of "fit" or with breakdowns in the individual's capacity to sustain her consciousness and action within what is recognized as real and rational.

Psychiatry and psychiatric organizations are concerned with bringing back order where it has been endangered by people who fail to sustain that version of the world which has been sanctioned as "reality". Sometimes this is done by reworking people through a variety of techniques so that what motivated the difficulty is removed or redirected; sometimes by intervening directly whether chemically or psychologically, to change the behaviour; sometimes by keeping people out of circulation until the troublesome behaviour stops; and of course if nothing else works, by simply stashing them away.

Though these effects are the same for men as for women, there is an important difference in the contexts which give them their determinate character. The psychiatric ideologies which justify methods of treatment and which interpret the behaviour of those as needing treatment, are part of the ideologies constructed by men from their perspective on the world.

Psychiatry becomes for women a mechanism of control which deals with problems of fit between the terms they are given to think and become conscious of their world, and the actualities of their experience. Psychiatry deals with the disjunctions between how women are supposed to feel and respond in their situation and how women actually do feel and respond and what their situation is in their experience. Psychiatry creates and authorizes for women ways of thinking about their unhappiness and despair, their sense of oppression, of being trapped by husband and children, or being stifled by subordination to the house.

Roles themselves are ideological. Women's role in contemporary society is not constructed from the intimate continuities of tradition. It is in large part taught, imaged and formed by the media and reinforced with reference to what is written, televised, represented in the movies. The role instructs us how to see events and behaviour as related to one another. It tells us how to put things together, how to interpret our own and others' behaviour. It tells us how to put together what someone is doing so that it makes sense in terms of her situation.

When what someone does or says appears causeless or senseless, this interpretive procedure has failed. It does not instruct us how the behaviour can be made sense of in terms of the individual's situation. For women, many of their feelings and experiences do not make sense for them and others in terms of the ideology of their role. The misery without cause, the unreasonable tears, the irrational behaviour – these all become visible and describable as such because the role doesn't provide us with instruction for how to see them making sense. They don't make sense in terms of the role. Psychiatry tells women as well as men to treat those feelings and behaviours which don't make sense in terms of the role as pathological.

Psychiatry inhibits the possibility of thinking these matters through to an alternative version of the situation. It deprives women of the opportunity of developing a language in which they can talk without shame – at least to each other – of what they feel and experience. The behaviour that doesn't fit is treated as a "symptom". As a "symptom" it is understood as pointing to the sickness of the individual. It cannot be related then to her situation.

Psychiatric ideologies take behaviour and situation apart and teach the patient and her family and friends to do this also. The patient must learn to understand herself in terms of sickness. She must address her past to find out what went wrong and where; to learn the causes of her failures to do what should be natural for her to do – to be a woman on men's terms in a wholly unnatural society.

The ways in which she struggles in the trap, the disjointed sentences in which she has begun to think herself through from where she is, the tentative experiments with a direction – these come themselves to be described as "symptoms". Lacking adequate formulation, they can have no direction, no outcome, no progressive movement. They abort at the outset. They become merely 'expressive', merely a motion or a gesture, a raving, a hysteria, an attack on the dark in the dark, a bellow of rage and anguish, a horror of not-being – that hole in the world through which its sense finally leaks away.[4]

Psychiatric ideologies refer such behaviours or assertions to problems in a woman's sexual identity. If there is something profoundly wrong with your relation to your situation which you experience as despair and misery, you learn from psychiatry to treat that as something profoundly wrong with yourself. You get what Pauline Bart describes as 'meta-depressions' – depressions in response to the experience of depression. She writes

> not only were we depressed, but we were depressed because we were depressed. Since according to the experts we suburban housewives should have been happy, contented, fulfilled and pregnant. What was wrong with us? [5]

In this vicious circle misery leads to a sense of not knowing where you are, who you are or where you can go. It is a circle which psychiatry creates. Psychiatric ideologies provide the instructions which connect women's experience of unhappiness in role contexts to emotional disorder. Corollary to this, is the view that the healthy or mature woman is at home and contented in her wifely and motherly role.

It is hardly surprising to find that married women go into psychotherapy a good deal more than married men.[6] Psychiatric ideologies interpret the world for women in such a way as to create a special demand for psychiatry, particularly among women of the middle- and upper-middle classes. If a middle-class married woman is unhappy she has learned, particularly if she has been to college, to recognize that unhappiness as her cue to go to the psychiatrist. She knows already that it is a sickness and that her obligations to her marriage and to her role require her to seek expert help for what is wrong with her. She needs fixing if she is sexually unresponsive. She needs help

 if she can't stand her children, if she weeps or is unaccountably tired, or feels constantly irritated by her husband. She needs treatment if she is depressed.

Resentment and despair are not treated as valid responses to her situation. The realities of her situation *as she feels them* are not treated as valid. For hers is not a special case. Her situation is 'normal' for our society. The difficulty which psychiatry reinforces is in seeing that the routine and sanctioned features of marriage and family can ordinarily and routinely give rise to such responses.

In psychiatric terms what is wrong is identified as what is wrong *with her*. There is no bound to the scrutiny of her self and her past which it sanctions. Her feelings, her past, her affections, her beliefs, her identifications ("did you ever feel that your mother didn't love you as a little girl?") are all in question. She does not know where to move in the world because she does not know what sort of world it is or who she is in it. Psychiatry instructs her to locate problems arising in her *relation* to her situation *inside* herself. Between what she knows most intimately as a matter of feeling and response and what is recognizable and sanctionable in terms of the ideology of her role, there is a gap. They do not correspond to one another. Psychiatry sanctions that disjunction. It places upon her the responsibility of learning how to live that disjunction as a permanent practice.

Psychiatric ideologies provide sanctioned procedures for attributing problems of the individual's relation to her situation to that individual as *her* problem. Thus the situation within which her anger and misery arises and which is constituted in those responses to it, can be peeled away from the officially and psychiatrically sanctioned realities of the role. What is normative authorizes the "objective" reality. The actuality which her feeling and responses began to locate must be discarded. Because she cannot act or exist in a reality which she cannot experience, the world becomes formless. She depends upon the psychiatrist to tell her what is there.

III

The position men hold in the apparatus governing our kind of society appears in the psychiatric relation as the authority of expert knowledge. But that authority is not a simple function of technical expertise. It is an authority which women do not appropriate. A study done in the United States by Phyllis Chesler[7] shows that the majority of women patients prefer male therapists and that the majority of male psychotherapists prefer women patients. The roles are apparently in closer congruence than the conjunction of women psychotherapists with male or female patients, or of male psychotherapists with male patients.

The reasons women give for preferring male psychotherapists are that they generally feel more comfortable with male therapists, and that they have more respect for, and confidence in, a man's competence and authority. This attitude is often accompanied by a specific distrust of women as authorities and as people. Chesler reports that both men and women in her sample said that they trusted and respected men as people and as authorities more than they did women. This appears to be the psychiatric refraction of the general relation of women as subservient to the ideological practices of governing appropriated by men.

Men represent to both men and women more than merely the authority of a special knowledge. They are invested also with the power and the authority of the institutionalized order of ruling of which psychiatry is a part. They appear thus in their professional contexts with an aura which draws upon the authority of their profession, and of the participation of their profession in the governance of our society. They do not appear in the psychiatric relation as themselves alone. Nor merely as the expert. They always appear representatively and always therefore in a borrowed glory.

The incapacities of women as authorities for themselves and for each other, which we can recognize again in Chesler's study of the psychiatric context, have nothing to do with fundamental competencies. They have to do with how women as a class are located outside the structures from which men derive authority. In denying women the possibility of speaking with authority women deny it also to themselves.[8]

Their own voices have no authority and cannot therefore voice their experience with authority. Women do not listen to women as authorities and therefore cannot treat what they themselves say as authoritative.

If we do not think of the term 'authority' merely as identifying an external source of commands, orders, advice, etc., but in a more primary way as identifying a social structure which assigns the authorship of acts, then to possess authority is to be that person who originates and appropriates the act as hers. Women's denial of authority to themselves deprives them of the capacity to author and authorize their own words and deeds. It deprives them of the right to complain, the right to originate knowledge, to recognize and declare to one another and perhaps to men, the reality which they knew if they had only known it.

Thus in the psychiatric relation they depend on the interpretations men give them. They learn to finger over their lives and to put together those shreds which will make the pattern they have been instructed to find in them. They have no opportunity to discover how it is shaped from within themselves or to tell it like it is. What is said in the psychiatric context by the patient (who is a woman) is deprived automatically of the character of authoritative speech. It is made over into a resource for the interpretative work of the psychotherapist. Understandings which might begin to formulate the actualities of their experience die in this relation before they can be begotten.

Women's denial of authority to one another conforms yet again to the denial of positions of authority to them by the world of men. Since as a class of persons they lack authority, they cannot be properly listened to. They cannot therefore get started on the work of thinking their situation through because they can have no confidence in what they have thought or their right to think it. Their interpretations need authoritative sanction before they can be taken seriously.

The role of psychiatric patient perfects this relation because the patient is always already discredited. No wonder male psychotherapists like female patients best. Women have already been carefully trained not to give credit to their own understanding. They have been trained to look to men to discover how to view themselves. Men don't listen to women, and women don't listen to one another. Male psychiatrists *hear* women in treatment, but women do not have the privilege of defining, categorizing, interpreting and assigning value to what they have said. That function is appropriated by men.

Where women are psychiatrists they have become so by virtue of learning to act in the professional mode from the perspective of men. That is a condition of being a professional. A woman who is recognized by others and by herself as properly professional is one who has learnt to think the world that way. Among the conditions of professional thinking in psychiatry, as in other social and psychological sciences, is a practice of detaching your own experienced knowledge of the world from the supposedly objective knowledge of your science. No leakage from the personal to the impersonal is permitted. The discipline is thus effectively sealed off from what women psychotherapists might know from their own position and experience as women. For that too must be reflected upon from the professional perspective. Thus the development of psychiatry as an extension of a male perspective upon the world has been scarcely modified by the handful of notable women thinkers in the field.

Freud explicates the strategy in a professional aside which appears in a paper discussing his theory of bisexuality. This theory links male and female with definite personality traits in such a way that they can be detached from the physiologically determined sex of the individual. Men may have feminine and women masculine characteristics. In the professional context, he points out, this theory has the special advantage of allaying the suspicion of women analysts

> that we, the men analysts, had never overcome certain deep-rooted prejudices against the feminine, and that consequently our investigations suffered from bias.[9]

They could be told that these 'unfavourable' views (which Freud does not repudiate) did not apply to the women analysts themselves. They could be told

> You are an exception, in this respect you are more masculine than feminine.[10]

The sex of the speaker is no longer relevant. It is the sex of her statements which counts. What women analysts might say from their experience as women is thereby discredited unless it accords with the perspective identified as male. Equating the "masculine" way of thinking with the professional or scientific preserves the hegemony of the male perspective on psychological realities. Women analysts are forced to sell out the rest of their sex, or be themselves discredited. As professionals they must locate themselves as men.

IV

The organization of the psychiatric profession itself preserves this general relation between men and women – the majority, the very great majority of psychiatrists are men; the majority of clinical psychologists are men; and the majority of social workers are women.[11] This hierarchical organization structures the psychiatrist's relation to the world and hence how he knows it. Those who govern and control do so in terms of abstracted conceptions of an actuality corresponding to that mode of symbolic action. The actual concrete and immediately experienced world is transposed for them into abstract forms of knowing. What actually happens can be known then in this form only indirectly and in the forms in which it is communicated.

In the health professions, as well as in others, the routine practices which mediate the actualities and transform them to correspond to the abstract forms under which they may be professionally (or "scientifically") known are performed largely by women. The words and concepts are the professionals' but they are given actual material embodiment by the secretaries who type them. The patient is indeed present as a whole person, but the routines which restrict the physician's relation to the patient and hence those aspects which come strictly within his professional focus are performed — in large part — by women: nurses, laboratory technicians, social workers, clerks, dieticians, and etc. The wives of professionals provide for the routine maintenance of their bodies and make available to them sexual services on demand. In various quite complex ways the world of the professional practitioner is organized so that he does not have to attend to its material actualities. He is sustained by a division of labour which accomplishes his abstract modes of action in its work of ordering, preparation, and realization. [12]

The anchoring of an abstractly conceived world in its concrete forms is not attended to because it is accomplished by someone else. That work is the less noticeable if it is performed by someone whose status silences them. Women are already silent. They have no authority to speak for and represent that actuality in its gross form nor for the work it represents.

In psychiatry it is the social workers who have direct and immediate contact with the uncleaned-up actual life situation of the patient, in all its complexity — just as anyone's life situation is always complex and rooted in others and other things and is not cleaned-up. It is the nature of the lived world to be that way. That actual life situation is where it all happens to the patient. Through her own work and the work of those who reconstruct it as a case history it is obliterated as it was experienced and lived.

By the time the patient gets to the psychiatrist she is already constituted as an abstraction. She has been separated from the contexts in which what she was saying and doing were connected. In psychotherapy she learns to practise this separation for she can bring with her into the office only what can be told. The setting she tells it in is his; the furnishings, the smells, the pictures, the drapes, the carpet, sustain the expressive order of the professional office. It constitutes a reality for this present which detaches it from other modes of being and gives present substance to an abstracted practice. In this place she will construct a biography, a social context, a set of problems, using procedures derived from the school of psychotherapy to which her psychiatrist belongs. The people in her life become the shadow people of the psychiatrist's office whose telling she works on together with him. Their reality as it is given them in this setting, and her reality in relation to them, awaits authorization in the interpretative practice of the therapist.

If she goes to a mental hospital, her personal effects will have been stored for the duration of her stay and are not accessible to her. Those which are returned to her for her use, as her clothes, etc., have been appropriated by the hospital storage and are portioned out to her routinely. She has been bathed, she has been cleaned up, as part of a process which Goffman calls 'mortification'.[13] In that place the people of her life do not exist even as shadows. They are simply in abeyance. She has been placed in a situation which is organized for her as an environment – fully external to her. She is an inmate and not a member. Her acts do not contribute to or become part of the work process of the hospital. She is its object, or rather its occasion.

Who she is begins and ends with herself. She is detached from her own biography as it inheres in the particularities of others' physical presences, in objects, in known settings, streets, her kitchen, *her* places. Her biography if she has one at all is one that could be told in any other way, that can be told again, and that dissolves into a fiction in the absence of its witnesses and survivors and of anchorage in concrete particulars. Her knowledge of herself becomes an abstraction. There is no opposition or tension between the reality she experiences and how it is named and interpreted. Everything is accessible to be conceived ideologically. The patient's own meanings and intentions are separated from the contexts in which they originated, and interpreted where they have no context other than ideological.

The psychiatrist encounters the patient as one whose abstraction has already been socially organized. For him also there is no war or tension between the realities he directly encounters in his working world and the ideologies he uses to name, interpret and order what he observes. He is not exposed to disjunctions between the nature of his psychiatric procedures and the actualities of his patients' lives. He is not exposed in his professional practice to the world prior to the practices of receptionists, nurses, secretaries, nurses' aides, and the patients themselves. They do a work which brings into being the forms in which what he does, thinks and says, make ordinary sense. His accomplishment of his role depends upon theirs in ways which his ideology does not permit him even to think.

The silences of women are complicit in the perpetuation of his abstracted practice. Their lack of authority to speak means that the concrete practices which abstract the patient from the actualities of her life are not represented. That she has no authority to speak either as patient or as woman means that she cannot represent her own existence. The rule that men do not listen to women is effective in this contact in the necessary silences upon which the practices of an ideological psychiatry depend. Psychiatry as it is practiced relies upon this relation of women; it relies upon women's lack of authority to speak; it relies upon their subservience to the abstracted modes of social control; it relies upon not knowing them and upon not listening to what they might have to say.

V

The women's movement in its varieties is relatively new. Maybe four or five years old depending upon where you are. But there has been a protest among women for many years and which goes back who knows how long and in what other forms in other societies.[14] So far as its psychiatric visibility is concerned, it has been going on for perhaps a century, perhaps for longer. Women have protested despite themselves by having 'nervous breakdowns', by becoming mentally ill, by suffering from depressions, by committing suicide (I remind you of well-known members of this protest, such as Charlotte Perkins Gilman, Zelda Fitzgerald, Sylvia Plath, Virginia Woolf[15] to represent the many who are not known to us by name). Women have protested with their lives. They 'took it out on themselves' because they could not do otherwise. They had no other means of acting upon and in their situation.

The psychiatric procedure for thinking the troubles of people puts a special kind of bracket around their behaviour by analyzing it as symptom. What women say about themselves from where they are is not treated as consequential when it is treated as symptomatic. It is not permitted to become an act or to participate in the construction of social reality. The social construction of behaviour as symptom takes the behaviour, so to speak, out of play. An episode in the TV series

All in the Family illustrates how treating behaviour as symptom invalidates it and prevents it from having significant consequences for the established structure of relations. In one episode Edith rebelled outright against Archie. I don't remember the details of the occasion, but I remember that she shouted at him as aggressively and rudely as he usually addresses her. The worm-woman turns at last, I said to myself, watching it. But her college-educated daughter put her back into place by carefully explaining to her that behaviour was caused by the menopause. Her action was interpreted in terms of the "change of life" rather than of her life-long subservience to a bully.

The procedure puts a special frame around her moment of rebellion. It tells us as well as the fictional Edith not to attend to it as an assertion about a situation or as having implications for how it should be changed.[14] Treating it as a symptom of her time of life sets it up so that others will not have to take it up on its own terms. In the setting of the serial drama it ensures that we will not be exposed to a disintegration of the relations upon which the series is based. The bully will stay bully; the worm will stay worm. The drama is again the paradigm of life. When next week's episode comes around, they will still be playing the same roles.

Psychiatry gives us ways of analyzing our protest which prevent us from recognizing and opposing directly the situations in which that protest arises. Symptoms are not produced by the patient, they are a way of dealing with what she says and does. They are produced by patient and psychiatrist in a joint work for which what the patient does or has done becomes the raw material. She offers the protest of her being for the psychiatric work of transforming it into the symptoms of a disease. It is a work of course which she may learn to do upon herself and in doing it she estranges herself further from her self.

The declarations women make about themselves are specifically invalidated. In one study of schizophrenic women, a patient is recorded as having said that she would go crazy if she was stuck with her household routines. And she was stuck with them. And she did go crazy. Her statement is included among an inventory of her symptoms.[16] By implication it is something that she will no longer say when she is better. It certainly cannot be treated as an account of what is wrong and what might be changed. It is more than her despair that is invalidated here. It is also her version of what is wrong that is deprived of authority. She may not even *think* the connection between her situation and her craziness. She may not offer an alternative account to the psychiatric version.

We did not of course recognize that this was protest. We did not know that that was what was happening. Because we had no means of thinking about what was happening as a protest, we went on doing it that way. In the women's movement we are beginning to discover our experience; to make it conscious and tellable and to invent for it the symbolic forms adequate to its representation. The other protest could not arrive at this because it was locked into the ineffectual and self-destructive iconic form of symptoms. As we become capable of speaking to one another of our condition, our relation to each other and to ourselves can be radically modified. In learning to speak our experience and situation, we insist upon our right to begin from where *we* are, to stand as subjects of our sentences and to hear one another as the authoritative speakers of our experience.

Notes:

1. See also Dorothy E. Smith, "Women, the Family and Corporate Capitalism," *Women in Canada*, ed. Marylee Stephenson. (new press, Toronto, 1973).

2. Simone de Beauvoir, *The Second Sex* (Bantam, New York, 1961). The formulation referred to here is found in her introduction to the book. It is the main analytical framework for the book as a whole.

3. See de Beauvoir, ibid., p. XVI-XIX.

4. In the first of his iconoclastic works on mental illness, *The Myth of Mental Illness* (Dell Publishing Company, New York, 1961), Thomas Szasz offers an account of symptoms as a 'protolanguage' in which people find modes of expressing what for whatever reason cannot be directly communicated in "conventional symbolic language". p. 299.

5. Pauline Bart, "Sexism in Social Science: From the Iron Cage to the Gilded Cage – The Perils of Pauline," *The Journal of Marriage and the Family*, November, 1971.

6. It is important to recognize what different rates of 'mental illness' among different social categories *do not* tell us. In chief, they *do not* tell us much if anything about varying rates of mental disturbance.

The point here is not that there is more mental illness among women than among men. This would be hard to establish. Partly because mental illness is fundamentally indeterminate as a phenomenon – how anyone decides that someone is mentally ill is not clear and the criteria are far from objective in most cases. Partly also because rates of treatment or hospitalization provide almost the sole reliable basis for estimates of rates of 'mental illness' in a given population and we know that these rates are determined by a variety of social factors having an indeterminate relation to the individual's state of mind and behaviour.

Here the argument is not that women's situation in society is more oppressive than the situation of men and therefore rates of mental illness among women are higher. I am not making any kind of casual inferences here. *It is simply observed that more women than men are in treatment*. More women than men come under the psychiatric jurisdiction as a means of dealing with their problems. The higher the social class and educational status of women, the greater the likelihood that she will seek and be able to pay for psychiatric help. If she has a college education she has had greater exposure to psychiatric ideologies and is more generally deferential to professional authority. She is more likely therefore to conceive her problems in these terms. The rates of treatment can in this context be read for what they do in fact show, namely differences as between men and women in the application of this form of social control.

7. Phyllis Chesler, "Patient and Patriarch: Women in the Psychotherapeutic Relationship", *Women in Sexist Society: Studies in Power and Powerlessness*. eds. V. Gornick and B. Moran. (Basic Books, New York, 1971), pp. 365-370.

8. This has been an important and I think crucial focus of political awareness in the women's movement. Chesler's study itself demonstrates the significance of this social effect in our society. Jo Freeman in a paper on "The Social Construction of the Second Sex", *Roles Women Play: Readings Towards Women's Liberation*. ed. M. Hoffaung Garskoff. (Brooks Cole Publishing Company, California, 1971) discusses women's prejudices against women. She cites a study by Goldberg which is particularly striking. Here is her description

> These distortions (of girl's perceptions) become so gross that, according to Goldberg, by the time girls reach college they have become prejudiced against women. He gave college girls sets of booklets containing six identical professional articles in traditional male, female and neutral fields. The articles were identical, but the names of the authors were not. For example, an article in one set would bear the name John T. McKay and in another set the same article would be authored by Joan T. McKay. Each booklet contained three articles by "women" and three by

> "men". Questions at the end of each article asked the students to rate the articles on value, persuasiveness and profundity and the authors on writing style and competence. The male authors fared better in every field, even such "feminine" areas as Art History and Dietetics. Goldberg concluded that "women are prejudiced against female professionals and regardless of the actual accomplishment of these professionals, will firmly refuse to recognize them as the equals of their male colleagues." p. 125

This study is reported in P.Goldberg, "Are Women Prejudiced against Women?" *Transaction, 28*, April, 1969.

9. Sigmund Freud, "The Psychology of Women," *New Introductory Lectures in Psychoanalysis* (Hogarth Press, London, 1946), p. 149.

10. Freud, ibid., p. 150.

11. W. Schofield, *Psychotherapy: The Purchase of Friendship* (Prentice-Hall, New Jersey, 1963).

12. See Dorothy E. Smith, "Women's Perspective as a Radical Critique of Sociology," *Sociological Inquiry, 44*, (1), January, 1974, for an elaboration of this phenomenon.

13. Erving Goffman, "Total Institutions," *Asylums: Essays on the Social Situation of Mental Patients and Other Inmates* (Doubleday-Anchor, New York, 1961).

14. Hysterical or self-destructive forms of action are probably much more general. They are, I believe, characteristics of behaviour in a trap and as such of course can be seen in both men and women. But in very many societies marriage is a trap for women and the nature of this trap shows in typical behaviours arising therefrom. Egan describes the ritual treatment of 'hysteria' among young married women in Ceylon. Here is a passage in which Johnson describes the trap and its consequences for Chinese women (in Hong Kong and Taiwan).

> If a woman was abused she had little recourse. Private citizens avoided going to the courts for help, so about all she could do was to go to her own relatives, who could put pressure on her husband's family. The meaning of this kind of helplessness has been made very real to me by one of my neighbours in the village where I lived in Hong Kong. She is a woman of about 55, who has been regularly and brutally beaten by her husband for the past 35 years. Even now, whenever he is drunk or needs money for gambling, he beats her. For a long time her brothers tried to intervene, but now they have given up and stay away. Her husband's kinsmen also tried to help, but now they have given up and just look the other way. Recourse to the police is not a viable alternative, so finally this year she went to the local temple to worship and ask the gods what could be done. To see a woman in this helpless situation is tragic. It

> was not uncommon for such desperate women to resort to suicide as their only escape, and incidentally, as a means of revenge, for public opinion would react very unfavorably against the people who had forced them to take this desperate step. Margery Wolf has done an analysis of the Taiwan suicide statistics from 1905-1945, and she found that the suicide rates for women, especially young women, were extraordinarily high as compared with those for other countries ("Women and Suicide in China," a paper prepared for a conference on "Women in Chinese Society," sponsored by the American Council of Learned Societies and the Social Science Research Council, San Francisco, June, 1973). In western countries the suicide rates for men are higher than those for women, but the reverse was true for Chinese women in Taiwan. She attributes this to the intolerable strain to which women were subjected in their domestic situation, one from which they had no escape.

E. Johnson, "Women in China." Unpublished paper presented at Chinese Festival, UBC, October, 1973.

15. Charlotte Perkins Gilman (1860-1935): American feminist writer. Author of *Women and Economics*. In a short novel *The Yellow Wallpaper*, she gives a vivid and horrifying account of the mental breakdown of a young married woman. She herself had suffered a breakdown shortly after her first marriage, intensified by the birth of her daughter in 1885. She lived the transformation from 'iconic' protest to overt political action. She left her husband, supported herself and her daughter by writing and lecturing and became an active feminist. She eventually married a second time but continued to live very independently and to be active politically. A brief account of her life can be found in Carl N. Egler's introduction to the Torchbook Edition of *Women and Economics: the Economic Factor Between Men and Women as a Factor in Social Evolution* (Harper and Row, New York, 1966).

Zelda Fitzgerald (1900-1948) was the wife of Scott Fitzgerald. She attempted in various ways to develop herself as an artist independently of her husband, particularly as a dancer. She suffered various breakdowns and eventually died in a fire in a rest home in which she had come to be an almost permanent patient. Nancy Milford has written her biography. Although Milford does not make a feminist analysis of her life and experience, the story she tells suggests that psychiatric treatment was used by Scott Fitzgerald and friends to repress her striving for autonomous identity and that her 'mental illness' was a product of her inability to suppress her will to achieve combined with continual discouragement and invalidation from those around her. (See Nancy Milford, *Zelda: A Biography* (Avon, New York, 1970).

Sylvia Plath (1932-1963). A major woman poet. She wrote one novel, *The Bell Jar* (Faber and Faber, London, 1966) which makes use of her own experience of mental breakdown and its 'treatment.' She committed suicide, having attempted to do so more than once. Her poem "Lady Lazarus," *Ariel*

(Faber and Faber, London, 1965) can be read as a statement of suicide as protest.

Virginia Woolf (1882-1941). English novelist, author of a very literate and effective analysis of the situation of women writers, *A Room of One's Own* (Nicholls and Company Limited, London, 1928). Quentin Bell has written her biography, *Virginia Woolf: A Biography* (Harcourt, Brace, Jovanovich Inc., New York, 1972). She suffered periodically recurrent cycles of manic-depression. These were closely linked to the rhythm of her artistic work. Her suicide followed the belief authorized by a physician with the encouragement of her husband, that she was finally and incurably insane. Her life, like that of Zelda Fitzgerald, still awaits a feminist analysis. Even Bell's biased account gives sufficient detail to suggest that her 'madness' was intimately linked with the contradictions experienced then (and now) by women who are artists.

I recommend for a feminist account of madness, Phyllis Chesler's *Women and Madness* (Doubleday and Company, Inc., New York, 1972). She discusses the lives and experiences of some of those I have mentioned here, as well as others, some of them among the many whose names we shall not know.

16. Harold Sampson, Sheldon L. Messinger, Robert D. Towne, *Schizophrenic Women: Studies in Marital Crisis* (Atherton Press, New York, 1964). This book documents, though not in these terms, the kinds of pressures to which women are exposed to conform to the role expectations of middle-class family living and how hospitalization is used to reinforce these expectations. The passage referred to in the text occurs in a description of the case of 'Kate White.' Since it epitomizes the process of treating failure to conform to role-expectations as facets of her psychiatric problem, I have quoted the passage in context.

> Kate, as we have noted, had been a tomboy. She was active, outspoken, and rebellious, a replica of her father. Marriage now made demands for heterosexual intimacy and emotional involvement, for more feminine participation in family life. She found herself unable to enjoy domestic roles or to perform them to her own satisfaction. She could not feel a sense of communality as a woman with her friends and neighbors. She could not fully transfer attachment from her father to a new man in a new family and felt increasingly alienated from her husband. Later, when she had children, she felt hopelessly tied down, frustrated in her career aspirations, and guilty about these feelings in relation to her daughters. *She felt she would 'go crazy' if confined to domestic routines.* Elements of sexual confusion and dissatisfaction with her role as a woman also found representation...in the recurrent idea that her husband was a homosexual. p. 55 (my emphasis).

The nascent protest in Kate White's actions and declarations are apparent. The passage referred to in the text of the paper has been italicized.

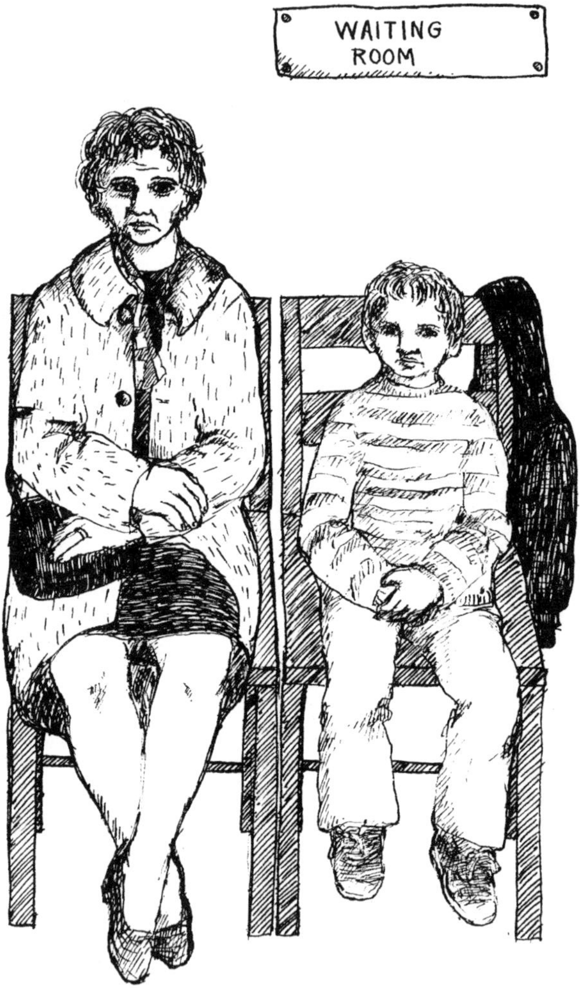
WAITING
ROOM

HOW THE PSYCHIATRIC PROFESSION VIEWS WOMEN

Elinore King

The kind of impact which psychiatric theory and practice has had on our cultural understanding and treatment of women has interested a number of writers. [Komarovsky (1953); Chesler (1972); Krakauer (1972); Broverman & Broverman (1970); Brown (1971); Rice & Rice (1973)].[1] The realization by these writers, and others, that the psychiatric profession has enormously influenced the situation women find themselves in today, reflects the growing awareness and critical exploration of the status of women. A closer look at the psychiatric literature, and at some of the ways in which the psychiatric profession views women, has important implications for increasing our understanding.

Sigmund Freud was one of the original contributors to describing the stereotype of woman, and this stereotype has remained largely unchanged in spite of the cultural changes since that time. How this stereotype is maintained and confirmed by present-day psychoanalysts and others in the medical profession will be described in this paper. It is important to understand how the stereotype implies that woman not only *is* a certain way, she is also *supposed* to be that way, and in all probability will *always* be that way. It is also important to look at how the psychiatrist views the woman who does not conform to the stereotype, and the resulting implications for her. This paper is an attempt to clarify some of the subtle ways in which prejudice reinforces and perpetuates itself.

When Freud defined the nature of women, he maintained that there was a biological basis for her particular make-up. Karen Horney and Clara Thompson, his contemporaries, attempted to show that women were the product of cultural, rather than biological influences, but at the same time their writings were largely ignored. Horney was finally dismissed in 1941 for her refusal to support the Freudian doctrine being taught at the New York Psychoanalytic Institute. Freud did, however, find support in the writings of two other women, Helene Deutsch and Jeanne Lampl-de-Groot, and perhaps the fact that they were female writers only gave Freud greater confidence in the accuracy of his theories. Deutsch essentially echoes his terminology. Hence have we inherited the 'stereotype' still currently prevalent.

The kinds of qualities ascribed to women are the following: – her "attraction to suffering" (Deutsch),[2] her unique ability to love, her capacity for intimacy and intuition in her relationships, her natural motherliness, – Besdine (1973)[3], says "motherhood should come naturally" – her especial relationship to her "inner bodily processes, " (Erikson),[4] her pleasing appearance, her sexual attractiveness, her "mystery" (Harding)[5] and her ability to perceive man as the strong and dominant sex.

More negatively, she is described as: – "masochistic," defined by Komarovsky (1953),[6] as "... an attitude toward life in which the individual uses weakness and dependency as a means of controlling others and of gaining safety in life," "narcissistic," that is, as a defensive reaction to the threat of her own masochism, she is illogical, incapable of justice, indecisive, weak, passive, dependent, submissive, jealous, tattling, manipulative, scheming, nagging, envious of men, compulsively feministic, and enticing. Whalen (1953),[7] categorizes women who marry alcoholic men into four types: "Suffering Susan," "Controlling Catherine," "Wavering Winnifred," and "Punitive Polly." Parsons and Fox (1960), state that a woman uses illness as a "compulsively feministic way of reacting to her exclusion from the life open to a man."[8] Kestenberg (1973), refers to "nagging" as the "typically feminine regressive way of dealing with internal excitement."[9] There are endless examples in the literature of such descriptions, which, both positive and negative, combine to form the 'stereotype.' The same descriptions are rarely given to men. These are the typical "feminine" qualities. Both positive and negative aspects of them reflect some of the ambivalence men feel toward women, namely that women have at once the capacity to be a mother or goddess, and also a scheming witch. All literature contains reference to this two-sided concept of woman, while the psychiatric profession tends to perpetuate the myth in a variety of ways.

While the stereotype of woman may not appear as desirable as that of man, with his qualities of courage, independence, leadership, and rationality, she is not encouraged to make any changes. It is legitimate for her to be envious of the man, but not to emulate him. In fact, any deviations from the norm of "femininity" are regarded with a good deal of disfavour, and are associated with underlying neurotic disturbance. It is not right for women to have man-like qualities, and the woman who does, or who deviates from her role of wife and mother in any way, is labelled in varying degrees, as pathogenic. Thus, it it legitimate for her to be "masochistic" or "compulsively feministic", but qualities of competitiveness, forcefulness, autonomy, assertiveness, disobedience, or pre-occupation with a career, are indications of malfunction. Lidz (1957), claims that marital "schism" and "skew", which may be responsible for schizophrenia in the offspring, are associated with confusion of roles in the marital partners. That is, if father is weak and ineffectual, while mother is competitive or domineering, their children will learn confused role-behaviour, and more damagingly, are likely candidates for neurosis or psychosis. Mothers thus described by Lidz are "preoccupied with a career," "consciously or unconsciously rivalrous with all men," refusing to "fill an expressive, supportive role" to the husband, and emotionally "unresponsive."[10] Usually she is breaking away from the socially acceptable norm, and more often, is simply adopting man-like qualities. Another description goes

> ... Mrs. N. was very sensitive lest her husband dominate her, and stood her ground with the help of a violent temper. She refused to accompany him on social engagements essential to his career and antagonized his friends. [11]

The fact that such a woman appears to have full use of her assertive faculties is a count against her. In such examples, one needs only substitute male pronouns for the female and reverse the roles as written, to understand the point. If this was a description of a man, there would be nothing "odd" about it, and Lidz might be hard put to suggest that such behaviour was damaging to others in the family, as in fact he has been able to do on the grounds that this is a woman he is describing. She is refusing to comply with her "wifely" role.

Lidz is not alone in suggesting that the woman who deviates from her feminine role is potentially damaging to herself and her family; he has, however, done much to substantiate the idea. Throughout the literature, the female who does not conform to the "stereotype" is labelled at least as abnormal. This alone might be tolerated, except that in her social position as wife and mother her abnormality becomes a matter of concern regarding the welfare of her family. She is, therefore, not only deviating from her role, but also held responsible for deviations in her family. Her responsibility is twofold – that is, she may be seen as the cause of what is wrong, or the potential cure for it. This heavy responsibility is not shared by the man in the same degree, as will become evident.

As a causative factor, the woman may be responsible for marital disharmony, as seen in the above examples of the dominating wife, or she may be unsatisfactory in her role as mother. Perhaps one of the most distressing implications for a woman is the probability that she will be held responsible for any mental disturbance in her child. If one of her children turns out to be a delinquent, neurotic, or psychotic, she may attribute this to her failure as a mother, which, in our society, is tantamount to saying that she has failed as a person. No similar emphasis has yet been placed on the father's role. There is, for instance, no male equivalent for "maternal deprivation," "the overprotective mother," or the "schizophrenogenic mother." This latter phrase became popular in the 1940's, related to the growing interest in childhood psychosis and autism. Some writers today still admit doubt in the area of autism, some claiming that no such entity exists. Nevertheless, descriptions of the "cold, unresponsive" mother still finds a place in the literature.

The schizophrenogenic mother:

Some of the definitions of the mother of the psychotic child include

> ...domineering, aggressive, married to quiet, ineffectual, withdrawn husbands whom they nag and despise, and with whom they are sexually frigid, [12]
>
> ...cold, rigorous, sadistically aggressive, [13]
>
> ...overanxious, obsessive, domineering, restrictive, perfectionistic, oversolicitous, dependent on approval by others, [14]
>
> ...emotionally detached and seeking gratification from intellectual sources rather than from contact with people, [15]
>
> ...sexually frigid...reluctant to have children [16]
>
> ...inadequate...compensating by making demands on the child in terms of her own patho-

> logical needs...defending against her anxieties by destroying the child,[17]
>
> ...much more involved in other pursuits, seeking her satisfactions and fulfillments outside the home,[18]

Such descriptions echo those early Freudian dissertations on "masculinity" and "penis envy," and Helene Deutsch's account of the intellectual woman, whose "warm, intuitive knowledge has yielded to cold, unproductive thinking."

The overprotective mother:

This particular description arose in the 1930's, again in relation to the etiology of disturbances in children. The "overprotective" mother is generally agreed to be as rejecting of her child as is the "depriving" mother: she simply shows her hostility in another way, namely by coddling, babying, fussing, and pampering the child until well into its teenage years. This is referred to as "covert" rejection, as opposed to the "overt" rejection of the schizophrenogenic mother. Again, there is a fairly wide generality of the type of maladjustment which can result from such mothering, including psychosis, or delinquency, Levy (1943).[19]

One of the important aspects of this area is that it is "fuzzy" – that is, there seems to be areas of incongruity or disparity in the descriptions of the "rejecting" mothers. It is, for instance, not clear whether they are dependent on other people or avoid them, whether they ignore their children or are oversolicitous, whether they are overly cold or whether they are overly loving. What seems to be happening is that the psychiatrist is seeking the cause, after the event has taken place. He first makes the assumption that there must be a fault in the mothering, since the child is abnormal, and describes the qualities of the mothers he interviews, basing the strength of his argument on the fact that they have characteristics in common. Since these qualities also correspond to Freudian descriptions of the "masculine" woman, together with all the implications that there is something wrong with that, the psychiatrist perhaps finds it easy to believe that a mother with such qualities must have a damaging effect on her child. Perhaps he also reacts negatively to these qualities himself. Fathers tend not to be looked at as critically, and in many instances assume the role of "victim" of the wife's domineering, for instance

> ...the husband withdraws from the relationship in an effort to *preserve some integrity* when *defeated* in the struggle, and may find *solace* in alcohol,[20]

It then follows that the psychiatrist will look for the same negative qualities in the next samples of mothers he interviews. If they happen to have rather different characteristics, – i.e. if some mothers turn out not to be "cold" at all, but, on the contrary, to be extremely loving, – he tells himself that this is merely the same quality under another guise. In the meantime, descriptions of the "normal" mother are sometimes so abstract, or so glowing, that they become almost meaningless. Besdine (1973), mentions that the qualities of a good mother may well be found in a good teacher, or a good analyst, which may be seen as a tall order for someone on such a different salary scale. Besdine, however, argues that "motherhood should come naturally." If not, the psychiatric profession has a number of categories in which it can place her, and will – she may be "negligent," "reluctant," "dedicated" (this has the negative definition of "pushiness," rather than the positive meaning which the word implies), and even a "Jocasta" mother. These alternatives all have the potential of damaging the child, although the Jocasta mother, through circumstances not altogether within her control it seems, may produce a genius, and has been flatteringly described as a "gardener" who tends her child like a rare plant in a hothouse.[21]

Another example of a lack of consistency in the literature is that it seems to be unclear whether or not there is love between the mother and her child. Some claim that this is the determining factor in the child's impaired development. Other writers, however, stress that there are strong bonds of love existing in the mother-child relationship, and that the child's impairment is in fact a bewildering phenomenon to his mother. Constructive ingredients in a relationship are sometimes hard to see, particularly by an outsider. Research favouring the mother-child bond as positive, has sometimes been criticized for being based on the mother's report of the situation. It is argued that the mother is not an unbiased person to be questioning about the relationship, and that she will, in any case, deny her hostility.

Such major discrepancies indicate on the one hand the dangers of subjective description, and on the other, the likelihood that the onlooker will find exactly what he expects to find. In more scientific circumstances, such descriptions would be classed as meaningless.

Another important factor which seems to have been overlooked in the research on "negligent" mothers is the possible effects of the interaction – that is, certain important aspects of the situation may influence the person being interviewed to respond in ways which may not be completely characteristic of him or her. Thus, the literature on school phobia tends to view the mother as a principal factor in her child's unresponsiveness to the school, particularly when she comes across as unco-operative, evasive, or critical. Whatever her behaviour, when she is under confrontation by a principal or teacher, perhaps in the school environment itself, it is usually assumed that this is her "nature." Little attention is paid to the possibility that she feels nervous and defensive about her position, and that her evasiveness, or her extreme permissive attitude, may reflect her natural wish to look good in a situation where she feels she may be blamed (and not without reason). In the same way, relatives of the mentally ill may be assessed on the basis of a conference interview, with little regard to the effects this particular situation may be having on their usual ways of behaving.

An example of some recent research which tends to ignore the interactional effects, and whose main purpose in addition is to confirm that there is something inherently wrong with mothers of psychotic children, is that of Goldfarb and his associates (1972)[22]. His research is part of a long study determining the effects of the mother's speech – based on volume, pitch, voice quality, rate, phrasing. fluency, stress, intonation, articulation, and communication of mood – on her schizophrenic child. The mothers who took part in the study were observed during a "surprise" visit to their children in the institution. The mothers were asked to visit on a certain day, which was not the usual visiting day, for the purposes of the study, and the children and mothers were then observed through one-way mirrors in a experimental room. The whole situation was strange, both for the mothers and their children, and was unexpected for both. The mothers were later asked whether they thought they were "behaving normally" with their child or not, and said that they were. Researchers apparently did not consider the possibility that their responses to the question might also be influenced by defensiveness, tremendous guilt feelings, or a wish to acquiesce in the face of a situation which involved so many implications. The behaviour with her child, noted by the observers, was

> ...passive, removed, vague, uninvolved...failing to maintain continuous flow of communication...

> failing to reinforce normal, acceptable speech communication.[23]

They also referred to "evasive, incongruent, illogical expression."[24] Never once is it considered that such behaviour might be the natural product of shyness, stage-fright, guilt, and bewilderment. No objective device was used to measure these qualities, which were simply judged to be "unequivocally outside the range of normal,"[25] by speech pathologists. The results of the study, of course, support the proposition that mothers of schizophrenic children tend to be unclear in their communication with their children, and with no other basis than this, the author concludes

> ...it is *presumed* that such lack of clarity is accompanied by deficiency in the mothers' regulation and orientation of the children.[26]

This research was accepted and published by a very reputable psychiatric journal, suggesting that where some subjects are concerned, at least, it is not too important to be scientific.

On the matter of subjective report, there are many descriptions of the schizophrenogenic mother as "sexually aloof," "frigid," or "emotionally cold." These words sound convincing, but it is important to understand that these are not "objectively measurable" terms, and that at best, the psychiatrist has only his own judgement to follow or perhaps the report of the husband who can hardly be said to be an "unbiased observer," and may easily be to blame for his wife's difficulties. If she appears "sexually aloof" to her psychiatrist, there are a number of reasons why this may displease him, and his judgement may therefore not be very "objective" either. The description of the cold, frigid, unresponsive woman is based entirely on emotional perceptions, and may bear no relation to reality. There are no measuring devices to back up the statement. For the mother of the disturbed child, their implication is highly destructive, particularly if she knows that she is considered, and in fact considers herself guilty.

Having examined some of the ways in which woman is the cause, or partial cause, of (a) marital disharmony, and (b) mental impairment in her child, it is now time to look at another aspect of her role as it is defined by psychiatrists – namely, that she has an important part to play as a curative agent. Some quotes from the literature on wives of alcoholics may illustrate the point

> ...a crucial variable in an alcoholic's prognosis is his wife's capacity appropriately to manage the marital difficulties consequent on his drinking behaviour, and this capacity may be determined *by personality factors*,[27]

> ...stability (of the marriage) is...achieved through the efforts of a woman who is *able to perceive her husband as masculine and independent* despite his obvious inadequacies, and *see herself as highly feminine and dependent*, notwithstanding the burdens and responsibilities of living with an alcoholic for many years,[28]

> ...it is a wife's *function* to accept her husband partly on his own terms and partly in terms of the concept of masculinity *endorsed by her social group*, and to make any of the social and emotional adjustments which follow from this acceptance,[29]

These prescriptions are simply an outgrowth of the concept of the "good wife" which Lidz and others refer to. It is the wife who conforms to the socially acceptable role who is able to save her husband from his own feelings of worthlessness. She must subdue her own assertiveness, in spite of the fact that she had to shoulder some of the burdens and responsibilities that a normally functioning husband would perform. The question never seems to be considered that she may have to submerge her total personality to do so. The most important factor is that she is the necessary element in the cure.

Similarly, women continue to be encouraged to take the responsibility for any sexual difficulties in marriage. An article by Peterson and Peterson (1973),[30] basing its arguments on a survey of modern sex manuals, describes how much more common it is for the woman, rather than the man, to be seen as the partner who can redeem the situation. Some of the more subtle implications in the manuals suggest that the problem was hers in the first place. As in the case of the alcoholics' wives, we are led to believe that her problem may have been to marry the man she did, whether she did so consciously or unconsciously. In this way, the woman receives no sympathy for her situation. She may be merely helped to remedy her lot by making some adjustments which will be more acceptable to her husband. Usually she will be "helped" to become better adapted to being a housewife and mother. Any feelings of resentment or anger at her situation will be explained to her as something she brought on herself, consciously or unconsciously, and thus any autonomy or strength in her will be discouraged. In the words of Krakauer (1972)

> ...her autonomy might be determined by the therapists' implication that she cannot make it on her own (needs a man) – and she will be encouraged to develop her sex appeal. [31]

Particularly in this aspect of "cure," there appears to be no equivalent role for the man to play. His responsibility as a curative agent is not as heavy, and he may receive considerably more sympathy for a disruptive home situation than a woman does. We do not hear of the husband having to "adjust" to the role of husband and father for the sake of his wife. Situations continue to exist in which a man will send his wife or girlfriend to a psychiatrist because she is refusing to take care of her physical appearance, or in other words, make herself attractive for him, Ellis, (1970).[32] This is apparently quite an acceptable situation, while it is hard to imagine how a male would react if his wife or girlfriend sent *him* to the psychiatrist for the purpose of making him more manly and aggressive.

The concept of female autonomy and assertiveness is discouraged by the psychiatric profession, and in some instances is actively ridiculed. Storr (1968),[33] claims that aggressiveness in the female is biologically different from that of the male. When a female attempts to be aggressive or dominates a man, there is something deeply shameful about it according to Storr, who believes that: "...ruthlessness in a man is admired," whereas in women, it is not. When she tries to assert herself,

> ...she becomes opinionated and dogmatic, and shows that insecure assertiveness *which men find tiresome* when they have to work for female executives. [34]

This discouragement of female assertiveness is a common theme in the literature, reflecting the general disfavour with which "man-like" qualities in women are regarded. Such a strong emphasis on women remaining in, and adjusting better to, the feminine role, has the function of excluding them from male intellectual practises and domains. It encourages them to remain in the home and retain their role of keeping the family fed, cared for, and in good health. From the psychiatric viewpoint, which is essentially male, there appear to be many good reasons to maintain the status quo.

Some of the recent psychiatric literature and theory, particularly that concerned with family therapy, is tending to emphasize that all members of the family are responsible for whatever happens *in* the family. Thus, the responsibility is shifting from the mother's shoulders onto the shoulders of everyone in her family. Even father, who hitherto has been more or less excluded from being involved in the mental or physical welfare of his family, mainly because he was usually out earning the money when the social worker called, is now requested to be present during the interviews. Although this seems to be a very positive step, from the point of view of women, a few notes of caution will be included.

1. Systems theory:

The concept of the "system" analogy in family therapy has been introduced as a useful means of observing and treating family interactions, the idea being that when one part of the system is operating in a certain way, the other parts will perform in certain other ways so as to maintain the status quo. When, for instance, one of the children becomes psychotic, this is usually interpreted as the result of a definite, if unspoken, decision on the part of all other members of the family that this should happen. The process is referred to as 'scapegoating'. When the child undergoes treatment alone and begins to recover, other members of his family will struggle to maintain the situation as it was – that is, to maintain the child's psychosis, often because the pressure is then taken off the family 'psychosis'. Treatment of the whole family at once, then, is a means of dealing with these situations as they occur. This analogy certainly has its uses, but may have its dangers too. In order to maintain the systems analogy, there is a concomitant emphasis on "functions" – that is, of each of the members of the family. Each is seen as having his or her function within the system. Since these functions refer to those tasks performed by people for the purpose of maintaining a situation, a certain depersonalization process is taking place. The process is still susceptible to the particular prejudice of the psychiatrist, who might for instance, see the wife's "function" as home-maker and mother, and may have little sympathy for her interests outside the family. He may also consider father's "function" to be that of bread-winner, like himself. Thus the theory is not free of the personal beliefs of the psychiatrist, although it has the merits of emphasizing shared responsibility. It is yet another instance of the role taking precedence over the person. The woman, then, may not feel that she is solely guilty of causing disturbance in her child, but may have somewhat different concerns that she has not been "functioning" as she should within her family system, and moreover, because the system is complex enough that, for a while at least, only the psychiatrists seem able to understand it, she may have a choice either to admit ignorance and do as she is told, or else to question what is going on and perhaps be told she is being obstructive.

2. The 'double-bind' theory:

Another recent theory which has emerged out of the research into family treatment is that of the 'double-bind'. This has long been thought to be an essential component in the development of schizophrenia, and was introduced by Bateson, Jackson and associates (1956),[35] from analysis of verbal communication having to do with conflicting messages occurring in the same treatment. That is, assuming that in human communication a single and simple message never occurs, the 'double-bind' concept refers to a pair or set of messages which occur together, closely related yet sharply incongruent, and presented in such a form that the receiver is seriously hindered from seeing the incongruence, or doing anything about it. As it stands, this concept has validity, and has proved valuable in observing and treating impaired family communications. In theory, too, these double messages can be given by any one member of the family to any other member – that is, father to mother, father to child, mother to child, and so on. In practice, though, most of the examples given in the psychiatric literature suggest that it is the mother, with her natural illogicality and confusion in thinking, who delivers the messages, either to her husband or to her child. Some classic examples given, for instance, are of the wife who says to her husband: "I want you to be the boss," thus ordering him to behave a certain way, and by her order suggesting that she is the boss, and not he, (Weakland 1962).[36] Another example is that of the mother saying to her child: "It's time to go, now," meanwhile holding him too tightly for him to move. Both these examples hint again at the apparent "victimization" of both husband and child, and at the illogical, yet potentially damaging, behaviour of the woman. Again, if the woman is lucky, she will understand what it is she is doing in terms of giving double messages, or acting in a confusing way, once the psychiatrist points this out to her. It is just as likely that she will take time to struggle with the unfamiliar concept, and in the meantime, feel the shame and guilt at (a) her lack of understanding, and (b) her failure as a wife and mother. In actuality, she herself is in a 'double-bind': for the messages she hears from the psychiatrist may be equally incongruent, namely, "you are adult enough to bear the responsibility for your family's disturbance," and "you are not adult enough to function without my interpretation and guidance." Or she may hear the messages: "You are a woman, thus an adult," with "you are a woman, thus a child."

3. Toward a female therapist:

Some writers are beginning to suggest that women find themselves female therapists, rather than male therapists, on the assumption that some of her concerns and feelings of worthlessness will be interpreted in the light of cultural influence, rather than being seen as pathological symptoms [Rice and Rice (1973); Krakauer (1972); Chesler (1972)].[37] Although this certainly is a move in a positive direction, it is still the case that many female psychiatrists share the same viewpoint about women as do male psychiatrists, and may therefore be of little help. It is interesting to note, in addition, that this idea has already met with resistance, and a female psychiatrist, Rebecca Goz (1973), comes across with these words of caution

> ...the request for a woman therapist by a woman patient is in some major form or other nearly always a *disguised request* by the patient to duplicate, review, reinstate, reenact, repair, and recreate some powerful unresolved tensions in her relationship with her mother. [38]

She cautions the therapist to be aware of the difficulties of this situation, and in doing so, lends the same old touch of condescension and total misunderstanding of the woman's predicament. Even if she does understand it, which one presumes she does, she shows little of the sympathy so much needed. Perhaps too few women psychiatrists have enough sympathy for the wife and mother who has not had the help to become autonomous herself.

4. Research:

Finally, one last, and already mentioned way in which the psychiatric profession attempts to maintain the status quo is through research. Much research, as in the example of the

Goldfarb study, makes the assumption that women, rather than men, are responsible for the family disturbance, and therefore tends to choose mothers, rather than fathers, as the subject of study. Some mention has been made in the literature that a study should be carried out on the influence of fathers, but little has been done until now. It is assumed that, because the mother spends more time with her child and has the task of raising him, that she will have the greater influence in his well-being or his maladjustment. Since psychiatrists are mainly interested in maladjustment, the chances are that she will be picked as a subject in research into psychosis, autism, or whatever, and that results are likely to confirm the already strong expectation that her influence is indeed harmful. There are strong suggestions in the literature that the mother is *too* influential and powerful a person in terms of the damage she may cause, and that she should be carefully watched.

More positively, the trend of therapy seems to be gradually moving away from making the responsibility all the woman's, and making it more of a group concern. The human potential movement also emphasizes assertiveness in women, and encourages expression of anger; in this movement, too, there seems to a more healthy distribution of female and male therapists, and who appear, at least to some extent, to be more than usually aware of their own prejudices. The psychiatrist frequently does not have this advantage. Culturally, more emphasis is being placed on the father as an important and influential member of the family, and although little has been done to examine his role very critically, there is more hope that this will happen. The psychiatric profession, meanwhile, is receiving considerably more scrutiny than it has perhaps had for a long time, and as more is written by people who have either been themselves victims of the institution, or who have good reason to be critical of it, the more hope there is that something will change for the better. In the meantime, the most important task for writers on the subject is to shed light on the prejudices, and help people to have a clearer understanding of how the system works the way it does.

This paper is an exploration of what psychiatric theory and practise does in terms of viewing, describing, and treating women. Psychiatrists, like most people, are subject to the cultural bias which encourages women to adopt and maintain a role of housewife and mother at the expense of developing her assertiveness and autonomy. Since the psychiatric profession has such a powerful influence, it tends to do much to perpetuate the situation as it would like it to be, and it is important to understand some of the ways in which this is done. As this paper has hopefully shown, certain words, examples, and research are used which suggest that any deviation on the part of the woman from her culturally acceptable role is potentially damaging not only to herself, but worse, to her family. Her husband is generally portrayed as the victim of her domineering and harmful manipulations, while she is held responsible for the disastrous consequences of her refusal to adapt to her role. In addition, although the recent trend in treatment tends to emphasize shared responsibilities, I have attempted to underline the need to examine some of the ways in which these theories work in practice. It is essential to look at the words which are used by psychiatrists to describe women, and how they often may be seen to be highly subjective in nature, and considerably open to interpretation. The stereotype of woman is reinforced again and again, while much of the literature is devoted to exploring and discussing the nature of motherhood, female sexuality, the frustrations of being a woman, and so on. The male does not receive such attention, either negatively or positively. It is as though he is a "given" in the situation, whereas woman is the *object* of his study. In fact, the theory and practice of psychiatry is based on male ideology, while the pathology is female. Every example substantiates this state of affairs. Woman may be a goddess, and a mystery, but she is also the demon-woman and witch, and her evil powers must be held in check. It looks as though the psychiatric profession has successfully managed, until now, to do just that.

Notes:

1. K.I. Broverman, D.M. Broverman, F.E. Clarkson, P.S. Rosenkratz, and S.R. Vogel, "Sex Role Stereotypes and Clinical Judgments of Mental Health," *Journal of Consulting and Clinical Psychology, 34,* (1), 1970.

J. Brown, Editorial in *The Radical Therapist* (Ballantine Books, New York, 1971).

P. Chesler, *Women and Madness* (Doubleday and Company, Inc., New York, 1972).

M. Komarovsky, *Women in Modern World: Their Education and Their Dilemmas* (Little, Brown, and Company, Boston, 1953).

A. Krakauer, "Woman's Body, Woman's Mind: A Good Therapist is Hard to Find," *Ms.*, 1, (4), October, 1972.

J. Rice and D. Rice, "Implications of the Women's Liberation Movement for Psychotherapy," *American Journal of Psychiatry, 130*, (2), 1973.

2. H. Deutsch, *The Psychology of Women:A Psychoanalytic Interpretation* (Grune and Stratton, New York, 1945).

3. M. Besdine, "Nurturing and Ego Development," *Psychoanalytic Review*, Spring, 1973.

4. E. Erikson, *Identity, Youth and Crisis* (W.W. Norton and Company, Inc., New York, 1968).

5. E. Harding, *Woman's Mysteries* (Putnam's Sons, New York, 1971).

6. M. Komarovsky, op. cit., p. 37.

7. T. Whalen, "Wives of Alcoholics: Four Types Observed in a Family Service Agency," *Quarterly Journal of Studies on Alcohol, 14*, 1953.

8. T. Parsons and R. Fox, "Illness, Therapy, and the Modern Urban American Family," *A Modern Introduction to the Family* (The Free Press, New York, 1968), p. 542.

9. J. Kestenberg, "Nagging, Spreading Excitement, Arguing," *International Journal of Psychoanalytic Psychotherapy, 2*, (3), 1973, p. 265.

10. T. Lidz, A. Cornelison, S. Fleck, D. Terry, "The Intrafamilial Environment of Schizophrenic Patients," *American Journal of Psychiatry, 114*, 1957, p. 245.

11. T. Lidz, ibid., p. 245.

12. S. Reichard and C. Tillman, "Patterns of Parent-Child Relationships in Schizophrenia," *Psychiatry, 13*, (2), 1950, p. 251.

13. L. Hadju-Gimes, "Contributions to the Etiology of Schizophrenia," *Psychoanalytic Review, 27*, 1940, p. 423.

14. T. Tietze, "A Study of Mothers of Schizophrenic Patients," *Psychiatry, 12*, (1), 1949, pp. 64, 65.

15. J.L. Despert, "The Genesis of Autistic Behaviour in Children," *American Journal of Orthopsychiatry, 21*, 1951, p. 339.

16. M. Ribble, Reply to J.L. Despert, in *American Journal of Orthopsychiatry, 21*, 1951, p. 349.

17. B. Karon, "The Resolution of Acute Schizophrenic Reactions:A Contribution to the Development of Non-Classical Psychotherapeutic Techniques," *Psychotherapy:Theory, Research and Practice, 2*, (3), 1973, p. 29.

18. M. Besdine, op. cit., p. 30.

19. D. Levy, *Maternal Overprotection* (Columbia University Press, New York, 1943).

20. T. Lidz, op. cit., p. 245.

21. M. Besdine, op. cit., pp. 19-43.

22. W. Goldfarb, D. Levy, D. Meyers, "The Mother Speaks to her Schizophrenic Child: Langauge in Childhood Shizophrenia," *Psychiatry, 35*, (3), 1972.

23. W. Goldfarb, ibid., p. 218.

24. W. Goldfarb, ibid., p. 218.

25. W. Goldfarb, ibid., p. 219.

26. W. Goldfarb, ibid., p. 226.

27. J. Rae, "The Influence of the Wives on the Treatment Outcome of Alcoholics: A Follow-up Study at Two Years," *British Journal of Psychiatry, 120*, 1972, p. 611.

28. J. Rae and J. Drewery, "Interpersonal Patterns in Alcoholic Marriages," *British Journal of Psychiatry, 120*, 1972, p. 620.

29. J. Rae and J. Drewery, ibid., p. 621.

30. G. Peterson and L. Peterson, "Sexism in the Treatment of Sexual Dysfunction," *The Family Co-ordinator*.

31. A. Krakauer, op. cit., p. 33.

32. A. Ellis, *A Guide to Rational Living* (Wilshire Book Company, U.S., 1970).

33. A. Storr, *Human Aggression* (Allen Lane, Penguin Press, London, 1968).

34. A. Storr, ibid., p. 57.

35. G. Bateson, D. Jackson, J. Haley, J. Weakland, "Toward a Theory of Schizophrenia," *Behavioral Sciences, 1*, 1963.

36. J. Weakland, "Family Therapy as a Research Arena," *Family Process, 1*, (1), 1962.

37. P. Chesler, op. cit.
A. Krakauer, op. cit.
J. Rice and D. Rice, op. cit.

38. R. Goz, "Women Patients and Women Therapists," *International Journal of Psychoanalytic Psychotherapy, 2*, (3), 1973, p. 299.

WOMEN'S OPPRESSION & PSYCHIATRIC OPPRESSION

Judi Chamberlin

There are two ways to analyze psychiatric "treatment" and institutionalization of women: from a feminist perspective or from a mental patients' liberation perspective. The supportive, developing ideology of the women's movement has encouraged thoughtful women toward a feminist analysis. Feminists have shown that psychiatrists, by using the cultural stereotypes of women against their female patients, have oppressed them *as women*. Such analyses are both valid and easily accepted into the overall feminist ideology.

A woman mental patient, in this view, is oppressed because she is a woman, and not because she is a mental patient. She is oppressed because she is a *woman* who has been defined as "mentally ill". The development of a mental patients' liberation ideology will allow a more complete understanding of the specific oppression of *mental patients* – both women and men – by psychiatry. Women patients are doubly oppressed; both as women and as mental patients.

Feminists who have written on the subject of psychiatric oppression have done so from an outside viewpoint – they have not been mental patients.[1] Of course, *all* women suffer from the psychiatric values that pervade our culture – as they suffer from all sexist values – but sexism is only one component of psychiatric oppression. The feminist analysis leaves the rest untouched.

Women who have been "successfully" psychotherapized or institutionalized have been "adjusted" to the traditional women's role. When such a woman later learns, through feminism, to see how she has been oppressed, the sexist component of her psychiatric experience looms large. Women who "need" to be properly socialized by psychiatric means are women who have failed to learn the more subtle lessons that succeed in instilling docility in the majority of women. The "lessons" as taught by psychiatry are far more blatant. Women in individual psychotherapy (usually middle to upper class) are taught that mental health consists of marriage and motherhood, or more recently, a suitably "feminine" career (teaching, social work, etc.). Women in mental institutions (usually lower class) are rewarded for wearing dresses and fixing their hair, and instructed in the rudiments of "successful" homemaking (à la Ladies Home Journal); "lessons" which are usually irrelevant to their lives. (Non-institutionalized poor women are indoctrinated into the homemaking myth largely through the advertising images with which they are bombarded).

Women who are struggling to define themselves as autonomous are trained, instead, to believe that their unhappiness comes from within; it is only a "symptom" of their "illness". The women's movement, which has accurately analyzed the main components of sexism, has found it fruitful to attempt to puncture the psychiatric myth, both by exposing the basic sexism of Freudianism,[2] and by exploring the active sexism that pervades actual psychiatric practice.[3] The fact remains that these are feminist analyses, and, I propose to show, are therefore incomplete, even as pertain to women. (They are certainly marginal to an understanding of the psychiatric oppression of men.)

Feminist anti-psychiatry writers are professional, middle-class women striving toward a non-sexist mental health system. Patient experiences may be quoted in their work, but the theoretical framework is developed by the feminist "expert". The mental patient is still silent. This, too, is a form of oppression, one that is probably unconscious on the part of these writers. My purpose is to bring this unconscious bias into the open, and to illustrate the necessity for an analysis of psychiatric oppression to be made by mental patients.

There has been much support given by the basically white and middle class feminist movement to non-white and non-middle-class women who have chosen to analyze their oppression primarily through a feminist perspective. Black, Puerto Rican, Chicano and poor white feminists are, of course, attractive to white middle-class feminists. The women's movement, however, has a political obligation to support as well women who have chosen to focus their activism on other forces that are directly oppressing them (for example, racism and capitalism). All politically active women struggling for liberation should have the support of feminist women.

Women who have been oppressed by psychiatry have not been oppressed only because they were women. Their strivings for autonomy have been thwarted by pressing them into the limited roles prescribed for them as women, *according to their class*. Upper-class women can fill the role of Lady Bountiful. Middle-class women are encouraged to be successful wife/

mothers first, careerists second (in women's jobs), *and* to feel guilty. Working class women, who have few options, are forcibly returned to the grim struggle for existence by the even more grim methods of psychiatric incarceration and electric shock. *All* women are told that to be nurturant and self-sacrificing is the true measure of their mental health. All these forms of oppression have in common that the woman is being returned to her proper economic role within the overall sex-role stereotype.

Feminist analysis has shown that women exist largely outside the money economy, but in roles necessary to support it. Women work without pay in the home, or join the workforce mainly to do boring work at low pay. Leisure-class women escape their own "women's work" by hiring working class women to do it for them – and thus have unlimited free time to spend at such diversions as charity or psychotherapy. Indeed, it is mainly these women who have the time and money to afford the private psychotherapy (particularly psychoanalysis) that has been so eloquently analyzed and denounced by feminists. I do not mean to deny that feminist writers have ignored the horror of the public mental hospital (where incarceration is more a function of being poor that being a woman), but it has been an abstract horror, because it has not been directly experienced by these women. Feminists especially should appreciate that the best analysis of oppression is made *by those who have been oppressed.*

The mental patients' liberation movement consists of women and men who have been victims of psychiatric oppression, and non-patients (many of them mental health professionals) who oppose psychiatric practices. The proper role of non-mental patients in this struggle is uncertain – with some groups admitting all comers as equal members, some placing limitations on the role of non-patient members, and some excluding them altogether. As the movement develops, this role must be clarified *by mental patient activists.* Since psychiatric victims tend to be lower class and well-schooled in "craziness", it is easy for the more articulate, middle class non-patients to take leadership positions in open-membership organizations. It is for these reasons that I, an ex-mental patient struggling against the system that has been the direct instrument of my own oppression, believe that the mental patients' liberation movement can be most effective when participation is limited to ex-patients. The proper role for dissatisfied professionals and other non-patients (including feminists) is to work for reform in the mental health field.

Freaking out is a way of rejecting the limited choices offered by society. Rather than choose among a series of undesirable alternatives, one makes a non-choice – the unfocussed rebellion of refusal. Because it is unfocussed, it is unarticulated. Psychiatric "treatment" consists of encouraging or forcing an acceptable choice and eliminating the alternative of making a non-choice, by making the consequences so unpleasant. Poor and Third World people are not even given a set of alternatives to choose from – their only option is to "choose" to conform.

Freaking out essentially consists of refusing to perform one's role, and making that choice known in non-criminal, socially unacceptable, and personally unsuccessful ways. A woman who stays in bed all day and won't do her housework, a man who cannot function at work, a student who draws back from the stereotyped career and life choices; none of them can state just why they are so unhappy. (Even if they could, there is no one to listen to this "unacceptable" message.) By defining them as "sick", psychiatrists (like any thought police) isolate socially dangerous trends and discredit them. What would happen to the social structure if too many people exercised non-choice? Psychiatry, by isolating and stigmatizing many who try, thus serves the status quo. It cannot be otherwise.

Whether the freaked-out person first seeks out "treatment" voluntarily or is taken by agents (such as his or her family or the police) to the psychiatrist or mental hospital, the goal of psychiatry is the same: to sort out those who are salvageable and return them to their roles, and to confine and degrade those who are not. Psychiatric incarceration is presented (accurately) to patients as so unpleasant that it is worth doing nearly anything in order to evade it. At the same time, it is mystified by being presented as medically necessary "treatment". This final "test" is, of course, reserved for those who are unwilling to act their proper social roles – people who must be seen (no matter how disorganized their mode of expression) as rebels, or, at the very least, as strikers against society. By putting the stamp of mental illness of such protesters, their position is officially discredited. Whatever germ of truth exists in their protests officially becomes only a *symptom*, one of many symptoms that manifests the person's (now "patient's") psychiatric illness.

There is a double mystification in this process of psychiatric labelling: both the patient and the public (specifically, the relatives and friends of the patient) are systematically confused, but in very different ways. The "patient's" refusal to take the proper role is defined as an illness. For the public, this serves the function of obscuring whatever meaningful elements the patient's protest contained, by including in the class of "symptoms" both the refusal and the usually bizarre ways in which the patient has been forced to express it. To the patient, psychiatric labelling is this and more – it is the clear warning of the real retribution such protest will elicit, unless the patient drops the protest and makes an *acceptable* role choice. Disguised as a *medical* process, the social control aspect has been successfully obscured from all concerned (probably including the vast majority of psychiatrists and ancillary personnel, who are comfortably maintained in the fiction that they are engaged in the commendable process of curing disease). Feminist mental health professionals have also been drawn in by this fiction.

Thus, to the patient, psychiatric labelling makes clear both that bizarre expression is forbidden, and that the doubts and questions which underlie it are forbidden as well. Not only must one cooperate, but one must stop questioning *why* one must cooperate. One must *want* to do what one *must* do.

Ex-patients routinely experience any feelings of dissatisfaction as indications that they are getting "sick" again. Since *everything* that they did when they were "sick" was labelled a "symptom", any new deviation can similarly be seen as a "symptom", both by the patient and by family and friends. If the patient is unfortunate enough to still be under psychiatric surveillance, this perception will be further reinforced. This is the means by which the social obligation is internalized and regulated. Since the psychiatric stigma persists for life, rebellious people are effectively crippled in their search for a satisfying existence. Only surrender wins psychiatric approval (as can be seen in any psychiatrist's assessment of his "successful" cases).

Mental patients' liberation means learning, as a group, to free ourselves from this psychiatric redefinition of the major concerns of our lives as illness, and to recognize the real and radical meaning of our protest. This is a process we must accomplish ourselves. A true understanding of our own oppression is hampered by the interference of others, no matter how mell-meaning. The proper role for non-mental patient feminists (or any politically active non-patients) in this struggle is one of external support. Women mental patient liberationists who choose to work politically with mental patient men are analogous to black or Chicano women who work politically with black or Chicano men in their respective liberation struggles. To condemn their sense of priorities is both non-sisterly and oppressive.

Feminist anti-psychiatry writers have proceeded as though the larger number of women mental patients negated the experience of oppression felt by male mental patients. Both male and female mental patients are the victims of oppression at the hands of psychiatry. In addition, women patients experience specifically sexist oppression by (usually male) psychiatrists. In their zeal to isolate the specifically sexist component of psychiatric "treatment", feminist critics have unwittingly ignored or continued other dehumanizing psychiatric practices. The *real* experts on the forms of psychiatric oppression, the mental patients who have suffered under it and struggled against it, are in the best position to provide a complete analysis. This becomes possible only in the context of a mental patients' liberation movement, a growing group identification, and a developing ideology.

Anti-psychiatric writers (both feminists and others) continue to perpetuate the stereotype that someone else must speak for the mental patient. This stereotype is inherently destructive. Mental patients are people whose self-confidence has been systematically attacked and whose expression has been systematically discredited. The anti-psychiatric "expert" is still an expert (with all the privileges that that implies), to whom mental patients have been forcibly taught to defer. Anti-psychiatric "experts" may believe that they have freed themselves from the objectification of mental patients which characterizes conventional psychiatry. However, the *only* true judges of this are mental patients, who know from direct experience how it feels to be on the receiving end of depersonalization. If mental patients feel contempt emanating from these "experts", then that attitude is there, no matter how strenuously the expert may deny it or claim it has been overcome. Mental patients recognize this bias (which has been termed both sane chauvinism and mentalism by the mental patients' liberation movement) as accurately as blacks detect racism or women detect sexism in those who deny they harbor such attitudes.

Denying sane chauvinism is not the answer, just as denying racism and sexism is not. All people (mental patients included) must recognize the privileges which the trappings of sanity bring, and struggle to overcome these tendencies in ourselves. It was not so long ago that the rumblings of women's dissatisfaction were dismissed by labelling dissatisfied women "neurotic" or "castrating", but psychiatry has retreated in the face of the women's liberation movement.

Women who have gotten the psychiatric enemy off their backs *must* realize that the shrinks are still firmly on our mental patients' – backs. Things *are* changing for women – at least for white, middle-class women. They have not yet begun to change for us. It will take the strong and united voices of mental patients joining together before changes will begin to happen.

The gains of feminism in numerous areas of North American life have been enormous, especially considering the short history of the women's liberation movement. However, decreasing the amount of overt sexism in psychiatric practice is not the same as eliminating psychiatric oppression. Whatever impact feminism has had on psychiatric practice (and it has been minimal, compared with feminist gains in other areas) psychiatric power is growing.

The community mental health movement, supported by millions of dollars of government funds and nearly the entire spectrum of mainstream political opinion, is not merely supplanting the old public hospital system, it is growing alongside it, vastly increasing the reach and power of psychiatry. Community mental health means more people will come in contact with psychiatric power – either to be "helped" or to be thrown on the public hospital scrap heap, out of sight (and out of the minds of those who are impressed with shiny new buildings and assume that everything is under control). We – mental patients – are ignored, or ridiculed, or made faceless once again by a new set of experts.

So, if you've never been forcibly numbed with Thorazine, if you've never had to wear old, shapeless clothes with X Public Hospital in letters three inches high across your back, if you've never been stripped of your clothes and your possessions and seen your world shrunken down to the confines of a locked ward – don't tell me about psychiatric oppression. Don't interview me or record my answers. Don't sympathize, or tell me that I'm all right now, or try to convince me that it's all in the past and it doesn't matter anyhow. It happened, and it matters, and I'm full of anger and bitterness that are an integral part of everything I have to say.

I was punished for questioning, for wondering, for trying to figure out who I was and what I should do and what it all meant. I still carry the scars of that experience. Every time I let an "expert" speak for me, I betray myself. And every time an "expert" assumes the right to speak for me, he – or she – betrays me.

Notes

1. The best known feminist analysis is Phyllis Chesler's, *Women and Madness* (Doubleday and Company, Inc., New York, 1972). Chesler is a psychologist. I have also examined two well-known feminist anthologies: *Woman in Sexist Society: Studies in Power and Powerlessness*. eds. V. Gornick and B. Moran. (Signet, New York, 1972); and, *Sisterhood is Powerful:An Anthology of Writings from the Woman's Liberation Movement*. ed. R. Morgan. (Vintage, New York, 1970). *Woman in Sexist Society*, contains six papers concerning psychology or psychiatry, all written by professionals: Margaret Adams (social worker), Judith M. Bardwick and Elizabeth Douvan (psychologists), Pauline B. Bart (sociologist), Jessie Bernard (sociologist), Phyllis Chesler and Naomi Weisstein (psychologists). *Sisterhood is Powerful*, contains three relevant papers: by Natalie Shainess (psychiatrist and psychoanalyst), Mary Jane Sherfey (psychiatrist), and Naomi Weisstein. Both anothologies are careful to include black women, Chicanas, and Lesbians as their own spokespeople. The *only* acknowledgement of the existence of the mental patients' liberation movement that I have been able to find in the feminist literature is *Vaginal Politics* (Quadrangle, New York, 1972), by Ellen Frankfort, who is a journalist, not a mental health professional.

2. See, for example, Betty Friedan, *The Feminine Mystique* (Dell Publishing Company, New York, 1963) and Kate Millet, *Sexual Politics* (Doubleday and Company, Inc., New York, 1970).

3. Phyllis Chesler, op. cit.

IT WAS AN EIGHTEENTH CENTURY HORROR SHOW!

as told to Marsha Enomoto

It is so strange now to realize that I was just having a good case of the existential horrors from finally waking up to how things were after being pretty naive and living on Vancouver Island and in the country. I'd been a student at University of British Columbia and the whole academic scene upset me, all those pseudo-intellectuals running around. It all seemed very false and phony to me. But at the same time, I believed that this was what I should be doing with my life. I should be finding out about some sort of truth, or something!

It was so idealistic! My head was in the clouds and I kept getting hit by hard, cold reality. The psychiatrist I was seeing was not into knowing why I was freaking out. It was like having a bad acid trip all the time. When I was down – really heavy, flashy bad stuff. I didn't have any of the friends I have now. I was living in dorms with these nice prissy little girls who were out to get a husband. They were all nice and sorority, and they gave me the idea that I was crazy because I didn't want to live their kind of life. Seeing a psychiatrist just reinforced the idea that I was crazy because I was seeing all this stuff, and there were no kindred spirits to talk to. If there had been someone to really talk to, all this wouldn't have happened.

I've seen about six psychiatrists in Vancouver, all men. The kinds of treatment they gave me were appalling. Lots of shock treatments. Lots of nice blanking out, waking up trying to remember my name, "What's my name?" When I came out, I couldn't talk. I saw these things that were people, and there were words in my head, but they wouldn't come out. Just like a zombie! I'd go in, get high, come back – not be able to talk. Such a frightening thing! I had absolutely no control. My tongue would be this heavy thing in my mouth, so heavy! Shock treatment was supposed to relieve my depression, but it never did. It made me more depressed. They knew it never worked, but they kept on shocking me. And lots of antidepressants, lots of medication. "Take this dear, this will make you feel better". But it never did! They never picked up on the fact that I was looking for something.

It was around 1965 when I first got into hospital. I was 23, very depressed and very suicidal, and I'd slashed my wrists. I was at Health Sciences Hospital in Vancouver and afterwards I didn't know what to do. There was no one to talk to, so I went home to Vancouver Island and was waiting to go into hospital there. I stayed at home and my mother was driving me quite out of my mind. I felt that even though I was really depressed, it would probably be better just to leave and come back to Vancouver. I said I was going to go but got quite frantic about leaving. My mom called the police and said I was in no shape to leave. The police were quite weird; they put me in jail overnight where I really went berserk – started throwing plates around and went quite mad. They put me in a straight jacket and tied me to the bed in the jail.

I don't relate to any of this anymore, but I remember feeling really trapped, and nobody understood what was happening to me. Next morning they brought me before some kind of kangaroo court and told me that they didn't know what to do with me since I was a mess. They decided to send me to Riverview Hospital for observation. (Riverview Hospital is the main provincial mental health facility for British Columbia).

My mother called the police because she was so out of it herself she didn't understand what was going on. She brought the police into it and I was put into the East Lawn Unit at Riverview which was like a jail itself, at least it was then.

Riverview was about the end of the world. It was an eighteenth century horror show. All the doors were locked and there was this "big nurse" in charge, this really fucked-over lady. I was put in with all these people who were really in bad shape. Just the shock of being there brought me somewhat to my senses and I felt, wow, I've got to get out of this place or I really will flip out for sure. So there I was with all these people pissing and shitting all over the place. I was pretty young, you know, and I tried to just stay by myself. The nurse came over, "Now, Miss B, you must get over and mix"...with this whole horror show. I said, "No, I'd rather stay by myself." But she insisted that I take part in the activities. I can't remember what the activities were, but I'd see all these people sitting, rocking and drooling, and I knew that I didn't want to get involved in those activities. So they took away my cigarettes. I'm a real addict and after a half-a-day I broke down and said I'd sit at the table with the other ladies if they'd let me smoke again.

I went to see the psychiatrist and he said, "You're here and you're under observation. You've been sent here by the RCMP in Duncan. We've been watching you for a couple of days and I don't really think there's much the matter with you but I want you to stay here till the end of the week for observation. I think you have a problem of losing your temper and being too easily stimulated."

He had this big rap of what he thought was wrong with me and I thought – right, sure, I'll agree, just let me out of here fast. He informed me, "I'm keeping you here till the end of the week, and if you're good, no freaking out, no temper tantrums, then I'll let you go." So I phoned my friends in Vancouver and said I thought it was going to be okay. It was really awful there, but I thought I'd be getting out on Saturday.

I was really good – I got up at six, made my bed, went daily to the barf palace where they served breakfast. I kept myself quite reserved, didn't get into the hospital too much – I was just a model patient. Everything was going fine, or so I thought, when Saturday came and I went to have my release papers signed by the psychiatrist. My friend Sandra was coming to pick me up. Everything seemed fine. But I waited and waited until it got to be about noon and no psychiatrist came. I went to the nurses' station and the "big nurse" was there.

Nurse: "What do you want?"

Me: "Well, I'm waiting for Dr. X to come and sign my release papers."

Nurse: "The doctor hasn't come in yet. You will just have to wait."

Me: "Okay, that's fine."

I waited and waited until it was just about the time that Sandra was going to come and get me. I thought I'd check once again to see if the doctor was delayed so I could phone Sandra and tell her to take it easy. I went in to the office for the second time.

Me: "Dr. X still not in?"

Nurse: "No, and he's not coming in today!"

Me: "Oh! What's happening? I'm supposed to be released today."

Nurse: "He's not coming in today and you're not being released today. This is just a test to see how you react to frustration."

Me: "What? What? You mean I'm not..."

Nurse: "No! You are being kept for observation for an indefinite period of time."

This just blew me right out because I'd talked to some women in there who had been under observation for the same sort of court thing. Their families had put them there. One woman had been there for five years with no recourse. (Since January 1974, involuntarily-committed patients in Riverview Hospital have access to a Review Panel where they can plea their case. See current British Columbian mental health legislation.) She was just stuck there and her psychiatrist was a real bastard. There were weird things happening in hospital – a German doctor was really putting through this Jewish girl. It was just – god – like a concentration camp. I felt, if I'm supposed to be crazy, then what is all this?

All these things were flashing through my head and frightening me. I'm here and this doctor is playing games with me too. Maybe I'm going to be stuck in here and I won't be able to handle it. Maybe I will really flip out.

I told the nurse that this was quite a shock to me and asked her for a sedative or tranquilizer. But the doctor hadn't decided if he was going to dope me up heavily or just watch me for a while "au naturel", so I wasn't allowed anything. In retrospect, I somehow understand the idea that people should be responsible for themselves. But I was a real mess and I couldn't. I went and sat in the waiting room and I was just steaming and frightened.

This weird woman came in. I was sitting there in this chair trying to keep a hold on myself and this woman came up, really out of it. She started slobbering on me and mauling me. That was just the final straw. I thought, god, years of this, maybe years of this. I'm too young for this!

I went over to this big potted plant, picked it up and heaved it against the wall. That was such a good release. Great! I felt so good. But as I sat there all these nurses came running out screaming, "She's really going wild!" They called on two orderlies from the men's ward who grabbed me. I was so confused and angry I told them to fuck off and leave me alone. I didn't realize how to play the game. I was really stupid about it.

They bustled me down the corridor to a padded cell. In front of this small square room with bars on the window and a padded door with an observation window in it, they told me to "strip". I was horrified. I didn't feel like taking off all my clothes in front of these ape-like orderlies with their knuckles dragging on the ground and their eyes goggling around. I asked them to let me undress in private but they refused. The orderlies came at me and started taking off my clothes. That was it! All these things were churning inside me and I just started fighting and kicking. One of the orderlies had his hand here under my chin and was bending me back while they ripped my clothes and pulled off my bra. It was definitely like being attacked by some wild animals. Another orderly had my head in a visc and I bit his hand. With a scream from this orderly, they all went berserk, thinking that I was the one who had turned into a raving beast. They threw me into the room with nothing on but a hospital gown – you know – one of those little backless things.

I could hear them outside the door though I couldn't see them. They were looking down at me through the observation window. I flattened myself against the door so they couldn't see me either. But they would open the door, and everytime they opened the door I would start screaming obscenities at them. I was pretty out of it! Oh god, what an ordeal! I was put in solitary because I was bad, but they had made me behave badly by confusing me and making me justifiably angry. I was put in solitary because I didn't understand the rules of the hospital game.

Now there was just the room and me – a tiled floor, no bed, nothing, just the window and a big black grate blasting hot air at me. Soon they came around with a big needle and I said, "I don't know if you've looked at my chart, but I happen to be very highly allergic to Largactyl. I break out in hives and I vomit and I get very very sick from it." But they ignored me, even though I was now trying to be very calm and reasonable. They gave me the needle and sure enough it was Largactyl, and I started retching, vomiting, and banging on the door. "Please, could I go to the bathroom? I'm really sick! Could I have some water or something?" But there was nobody to reply to me. By mealtime I was really sick, lying in a heap of vomit, when a hand appeared around the floor with a paper plate and a wooden spoon, and something that looked like more vomit on the plate.

It was so bizarre. I was by myself and I had nothing to do but lie there and think – I'm trapped, there's no way out, it's like the end of the world! I was very frightened. I was just so scared of what was going on. I can remember I would take the wooden spoon off the plate and break it up in tiny pieces and make sort of geometric designs on the tiles on the floor just to keep my mind occupied. The nurse would come in to take this plate away and she'd see what I was doing and she would sweep it out so that there was nothing left but me, and the room, and the hot air, and the vomiting.

I wasn't allowed out to go to the bathroom. I wasn't allowed out for anything. The psychiatrist came by on the second day, or maybe the third day, I can't remember. It was sort of a timeless thing. He asked me if I had learned my lesson. I was trying to be calm. I hadn't figured it out. I was mainly trying to show him that I was a perfectly reasonable human being.

Me: "If I'm here and I'm mentally ill, if I'm sick – then why am I supposed to be learning lessons? If I'm not sick, then why am I here in the first place?" I had some nice bit of logic worked out for him.

Psychiatrist: "Ah, obviously you haven't learned your lesson!"

He turned around and walked out. Two more days went by and he walked in again. By that time I had lost any vestiges of pride or humanity or anything. I was broken. I got down on my hands and knees, grabbing at his pant leg, and said, "Please let me out of here, please, I'll do anything, I'll be good!" I cried and screamed, but he didn't say anything. Once again he walked out. A little while later, I was let back into the big freak show with all these beautiful human beings rocking back and forth, drooling, and I was just so happy to see them. Oh Christ, it was like nothing on earth!

I didn't know what was happening – but I thought I was pretty much in there for good, or at least, until they thought I had "learned my lesson". So I wrote to my psychiatrist on Vancouver Island. He knew me quite well. I told him that I couldn't handle this place. He got some other doctors together and they went to the court in Duncan and got a release signed for me. They all testified that I was *sane*, that I was really *sane*, and that I shouldn't be kept in Riverview. I found out later from my psychiatrist on the Island that the Riverview psychiatrist had written on the release sheet that I be kept in Riverview for an indefinite period of time for observation. It was like being sprung from prison. And that was my great horror show!

I was very naive and very dependent on people then. I thought I could get help from the string of psychiatrists that I saw, and later on, from the hospital, instead of getting help from inside myself. It took me such a long time to realize that I had to find these things myself. I had to come to grips with reality, and work out my own thing. Finally, I met some really good people to talk to, who understood what I was saying.

After being pretty bad for about five or six years, now – and for the last three years of my life – I haven't had any freakouts. I have the normal up-and-down, yo-yo syndrome which I'll maybe always have – unless I become an enlightened super-being – but I've had nothing to do with hospitals or psychiatrists for a good long time.

STRUGGLING TO BE BORN
Judi Chamberlin

Was it purposeful or just force of circumstance? The world wasn't really conspiring to drive me crazy; it was just accident that loving parents, concerned educators and healing doctors had precisely that effect. Like the single soldier who claims that it's everyone else who is out of step, and just as ineffectually, so I struggled against everyone else's conception of what I was and what I should become.

The first enemy was education. Longing to escape the rote and regimentation, I retreated into daydream and fantasy. What would have been accepted in a dull child was heresy in a bright one (and didn't they have my IQ score to blind them to seeing the very real – and confused – child?). What I needed was the opportunity to wander, to adventure, to question, and to learn – but there were no free schools then, and the city was far too dangerous a place to roam freely. The choices were narrow: conformity, which brought a pain that must be hidden, or rebellion, to be spared the pain of the classroom, but gain condemnation in return. If I had had the opportunity to grope toward what I sensed I needed, perhaps I might have found it, but there were no alternatives for children.

Sometimes I conformed, went to school and suffered, sometimes I rebelled, refused, and suffered.

Adolescence added the further torment of sex. In the repressive late '50's, a time of rigidly stereotyped sex-roles, I both longed for and feared the attentions of boys, who were strangers, almost aliens. Once again, it seemed that any choice was only a choice of which pain I was to suffer.

My parents, only dimly sensing my agony (we did not speak of such things to one another), sent me to a psychiatrist. It seemed logical to them, loving me and wanting to ease my pain. It seemed logical to me as well, out of step for so many years, I now had powerful confirmation that the fault lay within me.

The choices were so limited. Continuing my education – voluntarily once high school was agonizingly completed, a job (and what kind of job for a woman, without a degree, with no training or experience), or salvation through love (and what an easy conclusion for a child of the '50's)?

In 1965, I married. Redemption, or so I thought, through the roles of wife and mother – at last, no longer out of step. In a few months I was pregnant, radiant, joyous, at last successful in a role. Then miscarriage – failure! – and collapse.

Again, a psychiatrist, this time a dispenser of magic pills. I came to his office, cried, was given a handful of multi-coloured goodies, went home, cried, and swallowed pills. He was puzzled that I was not "improving." He suggested hospitalization. Out of longing to end the pain (pain which I could not understand, for hadn't I – for once – done everything *right*); I agreed.

In March, 1966, I signed myself into the psychiatric ward of Mt. Sinai Hospital, seeking warmth, support and psychotherapy. In a manner that would later become familiar, the hospital's first act was to change my medication. Now disoriented as well as depressed, I moved through the hospital's program of occupational and recreational "therapy." The first lesson to the mental patient, repeated in varying forms in every hospital I was ever in: Behave! Conform! Never directly stated, but all too clear. It was the lesson of the first 21 years of my life repeated, by an institution of force, this time, since I had failed to learn the lesson as taught by more benevolent institutions,

I had entered the hospital in an attempt to find relief for the pain of living, and found, instead, that any attempt to show this pain to my "healers," so they could understand and help me, was swiftly met with repression. A good patient was one who swallowed the medication, followed the hospital routine, and indicated a willingness to "cope" with the life circumstances that had brought about hospitalization in the first place. Breaking out of the prison, "rebelling," was a symptom of one's illness. Conformity was mental health.

Discharged after two-and-a-half weeks, I went home to my prison. There was no women's movement to help me see that my cold and unrewarding marriage was a trap; I became convinced that since I saw it as a prison, I was still "crazy." So I tried to convince myself that I was lucky (didn't I have a "good" husband, a "nice" apartment?), and continued to cry.

The lesson was still unlearned. Despite all the authority figures who had failed in the past to entrust me with the secret of life (which I still believed they held and could somehow be persuaded to part with), I now decided psychiatrists were the ones with the mystical "answer." Nothing in my experience had given me the confidence to seek it within myself, the lonely, the out-of-step, the sick one. I returned to the hospital, desperate to be "helped." They had "no room," turned me away, sent me in a police ambulance to Bellevue.

Bellevue, childhood taunt, nightmare of the unknown, cold shiver in the dark. Was it once a hill, overlooking a beautiful expanse of water? An estate, perhaps, children playing on the lawn? The ugly buildings, crumbling, yet still strong, thick walls – but the name says that perhaps there was a time before the ugliness. I never saw it clearly; first, they took away my glasses.

Half-blind, I groped along the hallway to my bed, pointed out to me by a bored aide. I wanted her to lead me to it, I was afraid of falling or stumbling, but she only waved. It was night, beds everywhere, snores and moans. I tried to get up for a drink of water, was yelled back to bed.

My parents, horrified, made inquiries, pulled strings, with money they didn't have had me transferred to Gracie Square Hospital, a place where rich alcoholics dried out and rich psychotics were zapped at $50 a shock. Terrified, having seen the price of disobedience (for I had defied the psychiatrists by not resuming my role), I tried hard now to be "good." The carpeted floors and pastel walls showed me one of my choices; the vacant stares and shuffling gaits of the patients returning each morning from the shock room showed the other. Again, the lesson: Conformity, or Punishment!

Why was I so convinced there was some secret, if only I could persuade them to share it with me, that I was led continually back to the hospital and closer to danger? I watched, uncomprehending, how "normal" people moved without effort through the routines that seemed to me so deadly and stifling, and was sure that there *must* be a secret, which *they* shared, and from which *I* was excluded. Again and again, I risked the punishment of drugs, the threats of shock and continued confinement, desperate to find a way to continue to live. In the meaningless rituals of life, I saw only death. *And I wanted to live.*

I know now that my terror had a very real basis – it was not "crazy" after all, but a confirmation of my sanity. The rituals were meaningless, such "life" was truly death. Having moved all my life from role to role, sometimes dragged, sometimes all too willingly, I was making a desperate attempt to truly live for the first time. I was struggling to be born. And struggling alone – I was being forced towards death rather than life.

But, back then, convinced of my weakness, wrongness, and craziness, I could not believe that the answer lay within me. No one was trying to tell me of my strength; calling me crazy was confirmation that I was weak and powerless. If there had been someone to say, "Yes, go on, feel it, see it through to the end..."? (But this was not to happen for years.)

I left the shock shop unshocked. (How incredibly lucky I was! Patient in six hospitals, suffering from "depression" – the prime "indication " for shock – then labelled with the stigmatizing diagnoses of catatonic or chronic schizophrenia, and never "treated" with the wires and switches of ECT! How did I escape?) Terror had me truly immobilized by now. A move in any direction seemed certain to bring death or destruction. Start "functioning" again in a marriage in which I already defined myself as a failure? Or leave it and go back to – what? Or follow the vague stirrings of a mind I had been convinced was crazy? The only way to stay alive was to do nothing.

I turned again to the wisdom of my psychiatrist. Surely, somewhere, he had the answer. If only I would be good (but it didn't seem I was ever good enough), he would reveal to me the secret of life, the secret of normality. The next psychiatric "treatment" for me was the structured environment: a hospital where every moment of the patient's day was regulated with "therapeutic" purpose. It sounded like a way of staying alive.

But Hillside Hospital was a farce. Unknowing or uncaring of my fear of the death I thought was imminent, the staff proceeded to process me through its routine. The "structured environment" prescribed that I could make no phone calls or see no visitors until I "earned" those privileges, that I could not step out of my "cottage" without a staff member, that I must participate in the daily program that combined the worst features of school and summer camp. The fact that all these requirements and prohibitions terrified me concerned no one; it was something I must do, it was my therapy. I was facing the terror of my own death, and they wanted me to mold clay. I was taken into an expensively equipped wood-working shop and asked to guide a board past a moving saw – I screamed and fled in terror of slicing off an arm – I was uncooperative.

I now became desperate to leave the place I had been so eager to enter. (The procedure had been as complex and harrowing as a college admission.) My action had been toward life; instead, it seemed they were trying to crush the last bits of life in me. I used every means I could think of to convince them to let me leave: screams, tears, punches, logical argument. They could easily have "shipped" me. ("Shipped" was hospital slang for being committed to a state hospital.) Instead, they released me.

I was out in the dangerous world again. I slit my wrists. I entered the psychiatric ward of Montefiore Hospital. I was trying to stay alive.

I needed time, safety and support. For awhile, I was given at least the time and the safety. I began to breathe a little more easily, perhaps my death was not imminent after all. But psychiatry is never content to do nothing, to let time be the healer. I was put on tranquilizers again. I protested, argued, begged, and finally resorted to hiding the pills in my mouth and spitting them in the toilet. Uncooperative again. My safe place was no longer safe; I already knew that drugs bent my mind and increased the feeling that something awful was about to happen. I begged to be released, "No, you're too sick." I longed for someplace safe, quiet, warm, where I could grow whole again. Suddenly, doors that had been open were locked; I was forbidden to go outside even escorted. Panic – I knew that unless I found the mythical "safe place" I would die. Panic – I pounded at the locked door and screamed my desperation.

Uncooperative patients are punished. I was committed to Rockland State Hospital.

The lesson finally learned. Freedom was an illusion. Only cooperation brought life. That life seemed like a living death was a cruel joke. But it was better than the punishment of confinement and depersonalization. I promised to be "good." There was no escape.

But first I had to be sent to the state hospital, bear the indignities to mind and body, prove that I was truly docile, broken, "cured." Only then could I be set free, confirmed in the belief that to walk endlessly through the motions of a living death was truly life, happiness and health.

It would be years before I would once again risk the struggle of being born.

first published in *In a Nutshell*, newsletter of the Vancouver Mental Patients Association

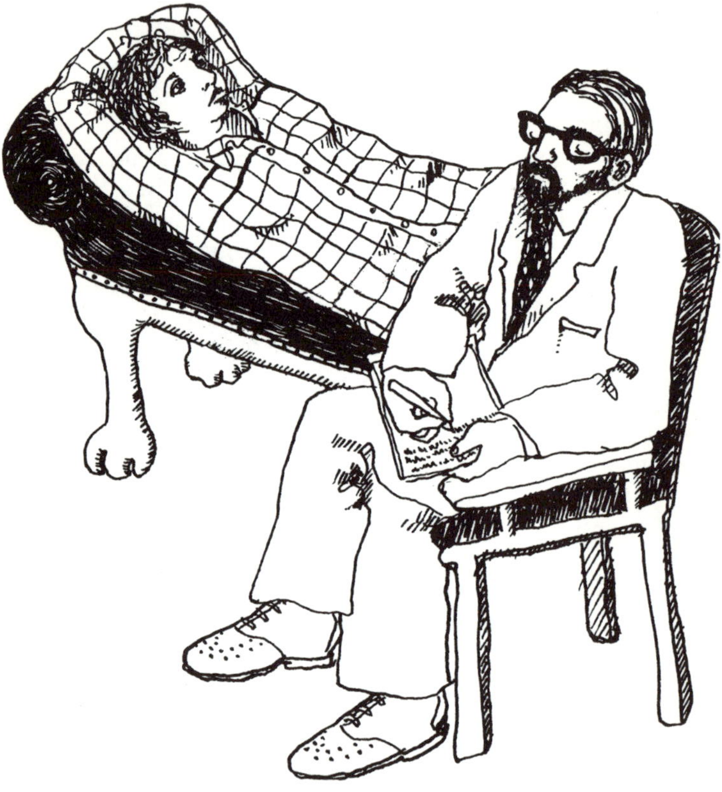

SHRINK! SHRANK! SHRIEK!

Barbara Findlay

I have been mentally ill. Hell, I've been psychotic, schizophrenic, manic-depressive – you name it. I have credentials as long as my arm certifying that I am an abnormal female, desperately in need of help to adjust to society and function in it "normally." The credentials aren't recent – the latest are now four years old. But if I were to return to a psychiatrist he would be pleased to update the diagnosis and pronounce me, if not outright insane, at least seriously ill.

I have done the whole trip – psychoanalysis, tranquilizers, suicide attempts, mental institutions. And the only surprising thing about it is that I emerged from it all still sane.

One day, after a particularly frustrating session, I asked the shrink, "What is the point of all this?" He answered, in tones of the greatest seriousness, "We want to make you into a normal twenty-one year old girl." I should have been warned!

I was always a screwed-up kid. In high school I was fat and brainy – a double jeopardy. I took a perverse pride in doing well at school, and I got fatter and fatter. As a result I was ostracized. I was weird, a freak, a teacher's pet, and I definitely wasn't socially eligible. But I couldn't have cared less. I wanted no part of the mating-dating scene. I found it humiliating to make a play for the boys. It made me feel cheap to dress and behave for their benefit. I considered the giggling-in-the-cloak-room, and the endless comparisons of past and potential dates by the other girls, to be ridiculous and stupid. I saw the girls as vacuous and almost contemptible. And so by choice I missed out on, never learned, the infinitely subtle social techniques that are passed on from generation to generation of adolescing girls in the pyjama parties and heart-to-hearts of high school.

Relating to the boys was largely impossible because of the heavy sexual underplay laid on any relationship. Essentially I had no friends. It was very hard for me to believe my version of the world – that the frothy parties and backseat necking were degrading and foolish – in the face of unanimous consensus to the contrary. When I looked at my face in the mirror, and heard the snickers when I got A's, I began to believe that I *was* a freak. I took refuge in books, and in endless frenetic activities – I was a YWCA leader, school editor, on the student government, a camp counsellor, etc. and forever. And I wondered why it was that all of those activities, which seemed so golden and appealing when I watched others doing them, turned into lonely tasks when I got into them.

I was desperately lonely in high school. I suffered from migraine headaches so severe that I was eating twenty or thirty aspirins a day. I thought, dreamed, fantasized about dying, leaving my body, somehow getting out of the world. I hated my incompetence in everything. My body didn't belong to me. I carted it around with me in a suitcase and plunked it down beside me wherever I had to go. I was invisible, and I was constantly amazed to hear people addressing the corpse beside me as if it were real. I fed the corpse lovingly, desperately, making it heavier and heavier to carry around. But it protected me from males, who ignored the mass of flesh and thus saved me from having to deal with the inauthenticities of coy sex games.

I had no one to talk to, to talk with, and so my unhappiness was secreted inside and I smiled brilliantly and performed wonderfully and wept at nights. Since there was no one to talk to, I became more and more isolated and more and more convinced that all the world was sane and happy except me.

From high school I went off to university. That I would go to university was a foregone conclusion. I chose one that was far away, would give me money to go there, and had a psychiatric facility (I checked the calendar carefully before I applied).

So there I was, just turned seventeen, all alone in a strange university. Like most other first year women I lived in residence. I was assigned a single room, which was unusual (most first year students must share rooms). And as it happened my room was geographically isolated from the "common room" of one floor, which made me an unwelcome interloper there. So there I was, knowing no one at university, virtually confined to the people in my residence and isolated even from them. And the few women I did know over meals or nearby me in residence were involved in the whirlwind of mating and dating – exactly what I'd rejected in high school. Such friendships as women formed were always contingent on their not being asked out. I didn't fit. But I couldn't even sustain my high school identity as a freak, because there was no one who knew me well enough to know or care that I was a freak. My isolation and loneliness, my inability to find anyone to talk with about things I now know are common to everyone, meant that the only reality for me was a psychiatric one.

It took me three weeks after I got there to work up the courage to find a shrink. I had no idea how to go about it – my information about psychiatrists came entirely from the doctor's column in *Ladies Home Journal*, and *I Never Promised You A Rose Garden*. All I had was a desperate faith that somehow a kind psychiatrist would make me "better". But the doctor's column had never told me how to start ("Hello, this is me and I'm crazy. Can I see a psychiatrist, please?") So I trundled off to see the Dean of Women, who didn't get alarmed at my misery until I told her that categories of reality didn't make sense to me: whereupon I had an appointment with one Student Health shrink for the next day. From that I learned what I had known instinctively: I had to talk about my life in recognizably psychiatric terms. With that began the psychiatric workup of my life that went on for the next four years.

I went to see Dr. Young (all names are fictional to protect the guilty) with absolute confidence in psychiatrists and their ability to help. Coupled with my faith in psychiatry was my conviction that somehow, my unhappiness was my own fault: that I was fundamentally wrong/sick. My head recited endless variations on "What's wrong with you?" "What more do you want?" "Think of all those people you're luckier than." "You narcissistic malingerer, you." (this last one only after I'd learned what narcissism was). I should have been happy, but I was miserable. Therefore there must be something wrong with me, I must be sick. Therefore I need someone to 'cure' me: ergo, a shrink. I had grown up in a Christian home where no one was mentally ill, they were just weak. So even to see myself as mentally ill instead of as a moral cripple was a major step and a great relief.

Dr. Young, as it turned out, was an orthodox Freudian, and I entered a treatment of 'intensive psychoanalysis' – the lying-down-on-the-couch, free association variety. He explained to me at the time that my problems were deep-seated and would require a long while to sort out, and that short-term psychotherapy (the sitting-up alternative) would be insufficient. This long-term treatment, he explained, was very expensive, and could be used only with a few selected patients with great potential for improvement. I went away convinced that I was very sick, just as I had suspected. What a relief! To be told that I was mentally ill was so wonderful, because then the problem was in me, and could be cured, and not out there – in which case I was doomed. I was also awed that such a massive investment was to be made in me, and I felt deeply grateful to be so privileged, to be one of the chosen few to be rescued from mental illness.

That "the problem" was in me, in my psyche or subconscious or id/ego/superego, was never doubted. All my contacts with the sundry shrinks I saw over those years began the same way, with an "assessment interview" to determine what my problem was, or what the diagnosis was. And what has always struck me about the intake interviews was the incongruence between what I was feeling and what they were asking me about. At first I took this to be official – my feelings that their questions were irrelevant was (obviously) further proof that I was sick... I made the mistake once, when I was admitted to the general hospital, of laughing when they asked me to count backwards from 10, and tell them the date and the year, and what the capital of Canada was. I laughed; and that was a fatal error – obviously proof of "inappropriate affect", and further proof that I was sick.

The first thing the shrinks wanted to know was who I was. And "who I was" meant: what do you do (I'm a student); how many siblings do you have (4 younger); parents alive and together (yes); and, inevitably, do you have a boyfriend (no). 'Do you have a boyfriend' in its various forms has caused me no end of trouble. I always failed that question, because I had never had a 'boyfriend' that I could produce as a talisman of my success as a woman. The shrinks always latched on to that gleefully as an important clue to my unhappiness (psychosis depending ...). In a tiresomely predictable way the questions went from there – have you ever had a boyfriend (yes); do you wish you had one now (not particularly)...And with the progression of questions I got into more and more trouble, because it was here that my version of life and their version of life diverged. For them, the fact that I did not have a man was a problem for me. And it didn't matter that I told them strenuously that it was not in fact a problem, since my vigorous denial was only further 'proof' of how much it mattered to me.

The shrinks had a corner on my reality. They were, after all, in the business of curing mentally ill people, and I was, after all, sick... Because I was mentally ill I had no credibility: they could believe my answers or not, as they chose. If my answers were wrong, I was denying the problem; if I disagreed with them

I was hostile and/or experiencing resistance to treatment.

It was a double bind with no out. If I refused to answer their questions I was resistant; if I told them it didn't matter I was denying. There was no way to convince them otherwise. Because they are the sane, normal, healers, and I was the insane, abnormal, sick patient. *They* got to decide what was true and real for me. And their job was to convince, persuade, seduce or threaten me to accept that reality as my own.

At the time, I did not see their version as wrong, but my version as wrong. I had a desperate faith in their ability to cure me: it was all I had left. And so I tried very hard to believe that what they said about me was true. I *believed* that I was merely hostile to, resisting, denying, my "true" problems.

I had two techniques to get out of the boyfriend bind. One was to answer all the questions matter of factly (are you a virgin? when did you lose your virginity? how do you feel about sex? are you sleeping with anyone now?) But that didn't usually work. My other technique was to lie. In the case of the missing boyfriend, I sometimes simply invented a conveniently absent lover. Such an invention (my distant friends would be appalled to know how they had figured in my psychiatric histories) worked in the short term (yes, I have a boyfriend but he is in Tahiti and leaving shortly for Timbuktu) but not for long, as my derangement was quickly ascribed to his absence. However, as a means of diverting the psychiatrist's attention from my missing boyfriend to me, and what I saw as immediately important, it was sometimes successful.

My lies were not dishonest. The truth — that the problem of whether or not I was established with a man, any man, a token man was not of paramount importance to me — was an unacceptable truth, and I had no way of convincing them that it was real. So what I had to do was present them with a version of my life such that they would see as problems what I saw as problems. Since I couldn't discount a lack of men as a problem directly, I had to present my life so that the problem wasn't there.

The shrinks were the ones who got to ask the questions. And I didn't get to ask questions back. So I had to learn to frame my life as a response to their questions. There didn't seem to be any holes in the situation in which I could wedge my version of my life. In choosing the questions they also restricted the range of answers. The simplest example is a yes-no question: if I say to you, 'I have a headache', and you ask

'Did you buy a new pair of shoes, I want to say 'No, but – but –'. Somehow the questions kept missing me. I still believed in the questions, though: the psychiatrist *knows*, and I don't – and so my feelings of frustration, of the irrelevance of the questions, was itself a problem of my resistance – and I also believed that.

In lying-down psychoanalysis of course there aren't supposed to be any questions. The shrink just sits behind your head and you are supposed to "free associate" – verbalize whatever thoughts, feelings, or ideas that come into your head, no matter how inane, trivial or irrelevant they seem to be. That was how Dr. Young and Dr. Duggan (the other psychoanalyst I saw after Dr. Young left) explained it to me. But it wasn't quite like that. Free associating was certainly something I'd never done before – talking at random to someone else for an hour with no replies is not something that is usually called for in everyday life. Some of my random verbalizations were "good" – they elicited "mmhmm – go on" from behind my head. Others got nothing but a dead silence. I began to realize that talk about my family, my sex life, and my relationships to the shrink were mother lode topics. At the end of an hour of such talk Dr. Young/Duggan would remark with satisfaction that it had been a good session. But talk about the question of human identity, or the white noise static in my head, or my terror of the shifting planes of reality, were disappointing, blocked. One time, when Dr. Young was particularly exasperated at my lack of free association, I determined to do what he wanted – to say exactly what came into my head. I did, and what came out were snippets of half-remembered poetry, random words that sounded nice in my head, a train of disconnected unrelated verbiage. Dr. Young was furious: I wasn't cooperating with the technique, I was resisting treatment... So 'free association' turned out to mean I could say anything I liked about priorly chosen topics. And he got to choose – though of course he never gave me a list – because whenever I started to talk about the things which made me ache with fear and despair, he would dismiss them as intellectualizing, and nonsense.

I remember one occasion when Dr. Young brought a book about some psychosis or other (I forget which one, now). He read me a long passage about some particular defense pattern (which I also forget) which blocked the patient's ability to free associate and then showed me where in the margin he had written my initials and the date, because I was such a perfect example of the psychosis... And on another occasion when I told the shrink that I had just won a prestigious scholarship, he was delighted. "You're the fourth patient of mine who has won that scholarship," he gloated. My achievements were somehow his accomplishments. I was being absorbed into his patterns of failure and success.

The question and answer frame and the free association 'technique' taught me how to do a psychiatric workup of my life. I learned that I wasn't despairing, I was 'depressed'; I wasn't angry, I was 'hostile'; I wasn't frustrated, I was suffering from 'free floating anxiety'. The whole vocabulary was one which put my emotions within me, and divorced them from the everyday world where they had their origins. At the time it didn't occur to me that my confusion and anger and unhappiness had anything to do with the world; it was my moral fault for not being happy in such a happy circumstance. Except that even the moral element was transformed in psychoanalysis: I wasn't morally wrong, I was mentally ill. Which was of course convenient because the shrink knew how to 'cure' mental illness. Psychoanalysis – four years of it – was a systematic obfuscation of the way I existed in the world. And I believed; I was a fervent convert to the myth, because since I saw myself as divorced from one world my only hope was to straighten out my id – work on my recalcitrant defense mechanisms – and have faith.

That is not to say that the shrinks had no effect on my life. Au contraire. The shrinks wielded an enormous power over me. When I was making decisions about my life, they would sometimes imply but more often state that one course of action would be psychic suicide, that if I did A or B I would go completely insane. They could sometimes enforce their views. Both Dr. Young and Dr. Duggan put me in psychiatric hospitals. They didn't commit me; they merely threatened to commit me if I didn't sign myself in. I went.

But there were other times. When I was entering my second year of university (after a year of Dr. Young's psychoanalysis) I had to choose a major for my B.A. I enrolled in honours psychology. The psychology department was heavily experimentally oriented, and clinical psychology was regarded as specious theorizing. Having gone through the registration hassles I went to see Dr. Young and announced my decision. He was horrified – first, because I hadn't consulted him in advance, but more because he said that for me to study psychology would be to jeopardize the success of my analysis.

When pressed, he explained that the view presented by the psychology department was in conflict with his own (Freudian) views; that the psychology department was wrong; and that if I got into studying psychology it would interfere with my successful indoctrination. He convinced me that to enroll in psychology was to seal my doom forever as a misguided psychotic child. Of course my wanting to study psychology was seen as merely a misguided hope of finding the answers to my problems in an experimental psychology course. Dr. Young also informed me that he had had to sign a letter of authorization to the registrar on my behalf, saying I was fit to return to school, and that he had been "sticking his neck out to do it". The implication was that if I persisted in studying psychology he couldn't answer for my sanity – and after all he had done for me to get me back into school it was hardly fair of me to wilfully endanger my (slim) chances of mental health. After a year of psychoanalysis I was convinced that I was sick. All my feelings, my problems, had been carefully severed from the everyday world and located in my troubled id, my turbulent ego, or my vindictive superego. So there I was, slopping around in a psychic quagmire: and my only hope was to *believe* that Dr. Young had the answers.

My journal at the time had this entry

Sept. 23/67

i've been trying to figure out what i'm going to do re subjects this year.

obviously my main concern is my mental health and therefore psychotherapy. unless i get my life unscrambled *nothing* is going to be of any use to me. and dr. young seems to feel very strongly that psychology just is *not* what i should be taking. so i should follow his advice – because he knows far better than i do what will be good for me. *on a rational basis* i realize that i should not go into psych for the simple reason that he thinks i shouldn't.

however, on an emotional level i balk at the idea. in the first place i find psychology interesting – statistics is even a challenge. social psychology would be fascinating, i'm sure...

right now my whole attitude is anti-switch, on an emotional level. on an intellectual level i am not as convinced of the magnitude of the problem as dr. young is – therefore i am merely accepting his word for it. so, in sum, it is my acceptance of his wisdom vs. my own desires.

Sept. 25

saw dr. young this afternoon – we decided that

i would take philosophy, politics, sociology and history.

It is amazing to me now that I could have been so incredibly trusting, so convinced that my salvation lay in Dr. Young's hands. But at one time my faith was the only hope I had. I was plainly very sick – we'd spent a year establishing that – and I couldn't possibly cope with all those newly-discovered blocks, my psychosis, by myself. I was ashamed of being mentally ill, coming as I did from a stiff-upper-lip Protestant home. So I never told anyone – least of all my family – that I was seeing a shrink. So the only version of my life that I heard was the one the shrinks gave me.

Dr. Young had a career all picked out for me. What I should be, he said, was a teacher of deaf children, because I had a warm and nurturant personality, and I would only be happy if I were helping other people. (I was a woman, right?) So I was all set to become a teacher of deaf children. He set up a trip to the regional school for the deaf with another woman that "I had to meet – she's just like you" – but the trip, like most of his other arrangements, fell through. And I thus escaped my nurturant destiny.

The next summer Dr. Young asked me if I would be his research assistant. I jumped at the opportunity, and arranged my life so that I could stay for the summer. I got a job working nights so I could work days for him, since I couldn't have afforded not to go home if I'd had only one job. Dr. Young set me up with a very nice fellow who was (he told me confidentially) also in therapy with him, and who he thought really needed to come out of himself socially and could I help? He put us together day after day with obviously trivial tasks, and great hopes for the outcome. But, much to his disappointment, Bill and I didn't strike up a flaming romance. I got a little edgy after the first six weeks or so wondering when we would be paid. It wasn't a topic I felt comfortable discussing during my analysis ("by the way, where's my money?"). Finally, when the end of the summer rolled around I asked him how much I should put down on my income tax statement as that salary. He said he didn't know, but I'd better just leave it off for the time being. We were never paid.

Dr. Young was leaving for another university that fall, and suggested that I switch universities in order to continue my analysis. He had such a hold over my life that I was convinced that unless I followed him, my saviour, I was doomed to insanity forever. I set all the wheels in motion but finally decided that that was rather too much, and stayed where I was – which was how I ended up with Dr. Duggan for the next two years.

Dr. Duggan was even less verbose, and even more conservative, than Dr. Young. He felt that I should lose weight and present myself in a more attractive manner. He told me that I chose unattractive clothes – my wardrobe was basic and practical, and there were no frills. He wanted me to date more often, to become involved with men. Looking back I discover that I disliked him intensely; but I didn't know that then. I paid a lot of money to see him, on the thrice-weekly visits he deemed necessary. He didn't feel that the medicare rates were adequate so he added a surcharge for each session. I was acutely aware, always, with all the shrinks, that I was buying their time. Whatever the rhetoric was, about a "good relationship" and so on, essentially I was buying their services. But that feature of the situation, like the rest of the real world, was studiously ignored. We all pretended that the therapeutic relationship was personal, not commercial. In reality, the boundaries of the relationship extended precisely to the end of the fifty minutes in each session and the capacities of my budget. I was supposed to put my life into the hands of the shrink, where it would be dealt with once or twice or three times weekly for fifty minutes, on condition that I didn't leak inconveniently into the rest of his life, so long as I or someone paid one bill. I ended up in hospital because I was beginning to leak. I was very concerned with death, which has always walked by my side the way some people walk with ambition. Camus said the only important philosophical question was suicide. He was right. I was wrestling with existentialism. It struck me as a true description of the world, but I could find no way out of its bleakness. And I was wretchedly unhappy and saw no hope for my life in any terms – philosophical, psychological, whatever. It didn't seem that it made much difference to the world in general whether I were dead or alive, and it seemed a good deal less trouble to be dead. Finally I got around to talking about suicide – a topic I had instinctively avoided. But suicides are not good for psychiatrists' reputations. And just as I began to trust, respectively, Drs. Young and Duggan enough, and when I became so desperate that I had no choice but to talk about suicide – precisely then was when I slipped over the limits of what could be handled in fifty minutes, and was put in hospital.

My first incarceration coincided with my first year university exams, which terrified me, and were largely responsible, in retrospect, for my panic. I had never seen myself as competent or bright – it was not true. The girl who went through school pulling down A's wasn't me; I didn't deserve the praise that went with the marks. I staunchly believed that every good mark was a fluke; I hadn't 'earned' it or deserved it, just somehow everyone had been taken in. So every good mark, every proof of achievement, did me in because I lost respect for the marker for being so obtuse that he didn't see how stupid I really was. I had no right to be competent – girls never do. So the first year exams were horrifying me, because I was sure I would finally be found out, and terrified of what would happen if I weren't. (I said once to a wise teacher "I'm afraid they're going to find me out" and he said merely "Don't worry; they never will")

I was so freaked by the impending exams that I couldn't face the world at all. I "slept" – a kind of unmoving stupor – fourteen or eighteen hours a day. And every time I woke up the pile of work was higher, and my terror was greater. On Good Friday Dr. Young decreed that I would have to be hospitalized. I trudged back to the residence from his office, explained to the only person who would have missed me that I had a strange sleeping disease, picked up every textbook I owned and walked alone to the hospital.

However it never occurred to me at the time that the exams were worrying me; I was just psychotic. And so I ended up in the psychiatric ward of the general hospital. The hospital was hideous. Since I was suicidal they put me on "constant observation" which meant that I was watched 24 hours a day by a ward aide who sat at the foot of my bed and read *True Confessions*. Every move that I made was "symptomatic" – a feature of my disease. They searched my belongings (but didn't find the razor blade in the cover of my French text). They read my poetry anthology while I was asleep, and the fact that many of the poems were "morbid" was a bad sign. They sifted through my garbage and picked up all the bits I'd written. I was naked and there was nowhere to go to escape their eyes.

Perhaps for me the worst part was having no credibility. The basic assumption of the hospital was not only that we – the patients – were "sick" but also that we were "unable to cope". Under that rationale they controlled every part of our life. And of course no one believed me – about anything. The golden truth about me carried no validity, and made no difference, unless it came from the lips of the shrink himself. My self no longer resided in my body, which was on public display in room 24, bed 1, but in a file folder accessible to everyone in the hospital but me. I had no way of knowing what was in the folder, whether it was true or false, compiled by a series of doctor's remarks and nurse's shift notes. But all the decisions which affected me – when I would be taken off "constant", whether I would be allowed outdoors, emanated mysteriously from that folder.

One day I got a letter from my last remaining high school friend, who didn't know where I was. She told me to fuck off, that she was tired of hearing from me, and so on. It was a vicious letter, but she couldn't have known. And it didn't do much for my morale – when they asked me why I was so upset I showed them the letter. And they didn't believe that she had written it: they thought I'd made it up myself. I had lost the envelope – and there was no way, I had no way, to make them believe it was not my own doing. There was no appeal from their version of my truth.

The only way to get out of that place was to convince them that I was sane. Pretty girl sane. I had to show up at the patient dances, make wallets in occupational therapy, be responsive in group therapy – the lot. There was no space to be angry, no way to criticise the hospital itself, because the hospital and everyone there was *obviously* there to make me "better" – and everything they did was "for my own good". So if I got frantic because I had no privacy – because, waking or sleeping, there was someone sitting by my bed watching me – that was hostility, resistance, a sign of my mental illness. When finally after eleven days and nights of watching it was decreed that I didn't need to be on "constant" any more and they left me alone for the first time, I pulled the curtains around my bed and sat underneath my bed – the only place there where there were no eyes. It was a fatal mistake; within an hour the watchers were back – I was obviously deranged, sitting under my bed with the curtains drawn.

But I learned also to be sweet sane. I have never been such a nice girl in my life. I dressed up, and did all those things I was expected to do, and finally they let me go.

The provincial institution, where Dr. Duggan sent me, was even worse. The wards were segregated and we had to go en masse to everything. We were not allowed to wear slacks to the dining hall – we had to dress up. In case, you understand, the standards fell. Constant observation was being in a glass room with six other people, and an aide at the door, who would dole out cigarettes and trips to the john one an hour. It was easier there to pass for sane; all I had to do was blend with the crowd and not make a fuss. And so my stay there was fairly short.

My only lapse was when I wept in the bathroom, and was discovered. They put me back in the constant observation room for that. The "rooms" had no walls to the corridor, and held up to twenty people. Always visible, always seen. But it was easy to get out of that hospital: put on a smile and a clean dress and you win.

There should be a way to explain how I got from there to here. I will never go back to psychiatrists, with their visions of sugarplums and motherhood. I don't really know what made me change. My fervent faith in the psychiatric version of my life just eroded slowly away, until I could no longer sustain the effort necessary to live in that made-up world.

In my last years at that university I had three very fine women friends, who were very important in making me see that at least I was not alone. Friendships with women were discounted by the shrinks as trivial. It never occurred to them that women had anything to say to each other or to learn from each other. I couldn't put together what I heard the women saying with what I heard the shrinks saying. But when I moved away at the end of the four years, and set myself up away from the shrinks' insidious influence, the credibility gap got greater and greater. I read *Sisterhood is Powerful*, and I was on my way to understanding what the psychiatric trip had been all about.

As a woman I am now much more at home in the world, because I see that the "fault", which I saw as my moral fault, was only the "fault" of having been born female. My guilt and fear of competence have dropped away.

The questions I was agonizing over – the meaning of life, and the question of suicide – have no answers; certainly not ones that can be bought from a shrink. But knowing that there are no answers I don't waste my time looking for them. To the question "Why go on living?" my answer is "Why not?"

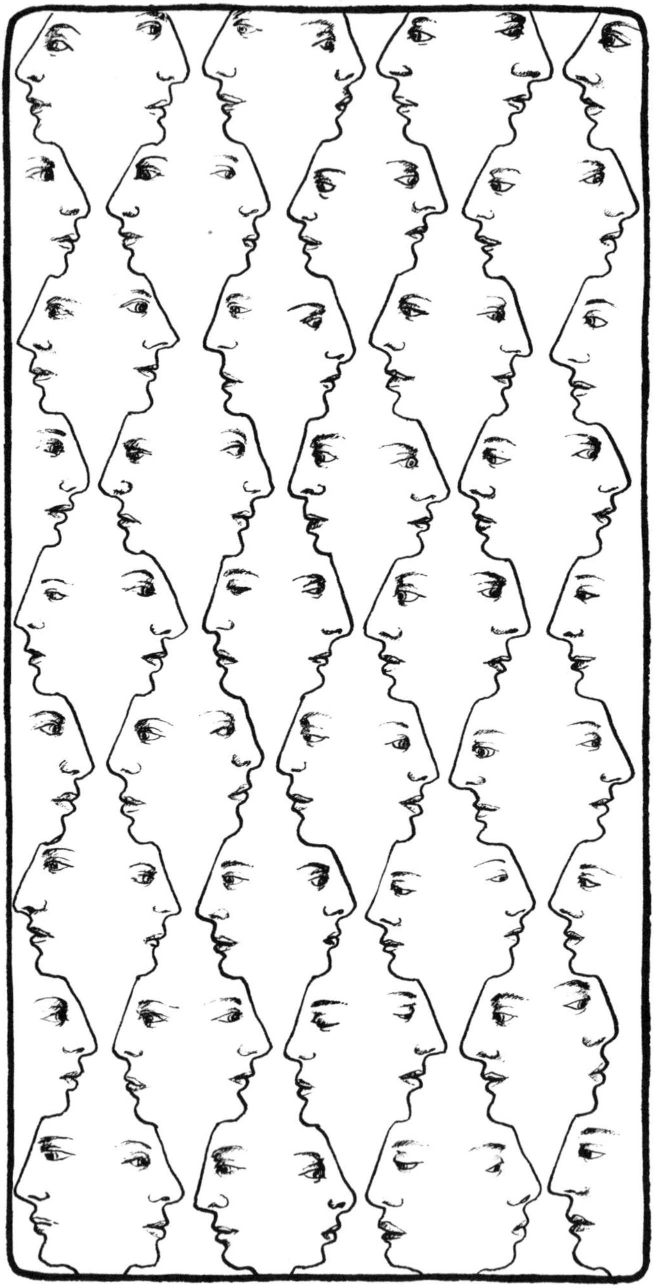

THE STATISTICS ON MENTAL ILLNESS: what they will not tell us about women and why

Dorothy E. Smith

I
INTRODUCTORY

This is partly about mental illness, partly about the Canadian statistics on mental illness, partly about problems of thinking about mental illness and partly about how to read statistics on mental illness. As you'll see these topics are less separate than they might seem. I've divided the paper up into five sections. This is the first and introductory section. The second is about what we want to find in the statistics and why it is that the Canadian figures don't show us the same kinds of relations between being a woman or a man and being mentally ill as some studies in the States have shown. The third section is about a problem in how we think about mental illness when we read the statistics this way. It is concerned with how psychiatry and psychiatric agencies of different sorts play a part in *creating* what gets counted as mental illness. As you'll see I hope, this is not quite the same as saying that psychiatry causes mental illness. But in any case it clearly makes for problems about reading the statistics. You end up asking whether anything can be said at all. The fourth section suggests a different way of looking at the statistics which begins by asking how the statistics get made and suggests that there is another way of thinking about what they mean and that it tells you something different about the process by which people come to be classified as mentally ill. And finally, in the fifth section, using this kind of approach, we'll look at some of the Canadian statistics, trying to see how they might happen and appear as they do and what we can learn from them. And further than that, what other kinds of questions are raised that we'd like to know about.

I've separated the sections quite clearly and tried to make them hold together internally. If you aren't much into reading about statistics or if you find the kinds of thinking presented in sections three and four difficult, then you can skip them. In fact you can pretty much pick and choose about where to begin and what to use.

I've only used the simplest and most obvious statistical resources. First from *Statistics Canada* (you'll find the references at the end of the paper) and then some B.C. Statistics. I haven't tried to produce an overall picture of the relation between sex and mental illness for Canada. There is some information here which you can use. But I think it is more important for the reader to know something about how such statistical information can be interpreted. Mental illness gives special difficulties in this respect.

It would be possible to do a much much more comprehensive study by making use of the provincial data as well as the federal. The limitations of the information given here are straightforward limitations of time and money. The work had to be fitted in with my job, etc. There was no money. These are real and ordinary conditions to any work of this kind. I mention them not to excuse, but to remind you that *these are the conditions*. By convention we represent our work as if it were done independently of the ordinary and necessary conditions of its doing. It's good to keep in mind that the material conditions of its doing enter into what is done. Particularly since those available for work that concerns women have been less than generous.

After you've read this you might like to go and see what is available, for example, on Ontario. If you do, I suggest you take along one of those little electronic calculators. There's no problem locating the sources, and librarians are very helpful if you get stuck.

In using the statistical material I've adapted it in some ways. The main things I've done are these:

1. I've eliminated certain categories of people from the figures – children under 15 and women and men over 59 (except with the B.C. statistics which doesn't allow us to do the latter). The situations of these people are distinctive both in the ways in which they may become mentally ill (older people are much more likely to experience organic problems, for example); and how they come within the psychiatric jurisdiction. The baseline I've used is close to that which defines the Labour Force on the dimension of age. Therefore the

tables I've presented here differ from the originals. The numbers of people in these age groups have been deducted from the sub-categories and totals. (I've had to use the figures for 15-69 in the B.C. statistics because they are bunched in such a way as to leave you no alternative.)

2. Since we are concerned with the interchange between social context and psychiatric forms of social control, I have also excluded where I can those diagnostic categories clearly identifying an organic cause. Organic illnesses also generally have determinate social contexts but their course, origin and hence the problems of investigating this relation are quite different. They are not the topic here.

3. I've also simply percentaged some of the figures rather than reproducing whole tables. This is because I have wanted to focus on a particular comparison. The raw figures are there, in the original and I've turned them into percentages to show, for example, the relative shares of women and men in a particular total.

I know that a lot of the reasoning here and the kind of information I'm writing about turns people off. There's a problem here because people also use this kind of information very casually. People depend on the experts too much. What often happens is that someone who is identified as an expert makes a statement like "the figures show a consistently larger female than male involvement with psychiatry." This is backed up with a dense array of numerical description. If you freak out at the numerical description you don't read it. Yet somehow its very presence adds weight to the statement. If you haven't read it, its support is mainly in giving the appearance of expertise. It *looks* like evidence, but you don't know whether it is. Then we go away treasuring this statement – which has probably shifted to 'So and So *has shown* that more women than men are mentally ill.' By this time we are a long way away from the real world but much, much closer to the world where we feel it's at and the world that we construct in talk with other women.

Part of what I want to do here is to make it as plain as I can how these kinds of things get done. I want to demystify the statistics. It isn't very exciting for the most part, but I think we should take greater responsibility for knowing how to look at the evidence. And mental illness gives all kinds of special trouble.

II

Do more women than men become mentally ill? Two U.S. studies reviewed and compared with the Canadian statistics.

We have an intimate insider's sense of a relation between powerlessness and mental illness. We expect to be able to see in the statistical information on mental illness evidence of the effect of oppression on women. We expect to find that the rates of mental illness among women are higher than the rates of mental illness among men. Proportionate to their numbers in the population (which at the ages we're concerned with is more or less equal), more women than men should be showing up for treatment or other kinds of psychiatric care because of this effect and hence get counted and show up in the official statistics – the social book-keeping of the nation.

This is Phyllis Chesler's argument in her book *Women and Madness*.[1] In Chapter Four she reports that a number of surveys which involve asking people questions about themselves show higher rates of mental disturbance or mental disorder among the women who respond. Some of what I'll say later raises questions about this type of evidence, but we are just going to be concerned with what the *official* statistics tell us. According to Chesler, the official statistics on mental illness in the States show

> a consistently large female involvement with psychiatry in America, an involvement that has been increasing rather dramatically since 1964. The total number of women in psychiatric facilities (including the predominantly all-male Veterans Administration psychiatric facilities) increased from 479,167 in 1964 to 615,112 in 1968. In 1964, there were 1079 more women than men in psychiatric facilities. By 1968, 50,363 more women than men were psychiatrically hospitalized and publicly treated (see Tables 4 and 5). During the 1960s, adult women, far more than adult men, constituted the majority of patients in general psychiatric wards, private hospitals, public outpatient clinics, and community mental health centres. In 1968, for example, adult women comprised 60 per cent of the patients in general psychiatric wards, 61 per cent of the population in private hospitals, and 62 per cent of the population in out-patient clinics. In 1968, women of all ages comprised 50 per cent of the population in state and county hospitals. From 1964 through 1968, 125,351 more women than

men were patients in all psychiatric institutions. Between 1950 and 1968, 223,268 more women than men (many of them "old" women), were confined in state and county hospitals.[2]
(the references to tables in brackets are to the tables which appear in the appendix of *Women and Madness*)

This adds up to a pretty powerful picture.

When we look at the Canadian statistics in their 'raw' form, however, we don't find quite the same relationship.

This information is for 1970 only (other differences from Chesler are noted below).

TABLE 1

Type of institution, first admissions, 1970, percent women & men (ages 15-59), *Statistics Canada*

	Percent women	Percent men	Total
Public Mental Hospitals	39 (4,608)	61 (7,223)	100 (11,831)
Public Psychiatric Units	60 (11,948)	40 (7,815)	100 (19,769)
Psychiatric Hospitals	47 (2,485)	53 (2,752)	100 (5,237)
Federal Psychiatric Hospitals	0.3 (19)	99.7 (709)	100 (728)
Hospitals for Addicts	21 (846)	79 (3,164)	100 (4,010)
All Facilities	48 (19,906)	52 (21,663)	100 (41,569)

Note: Numbers appear in brackets below percentages.

Here we are looking at in-patient services only and over a slightly different range of facilities (Chesler includes VA out-patient, excludes hospitals for addicts).

Public Mental Hospitals take in all kinds of psychiatric problems and include long-term care facilities and special "security" situations. Public Psychiatric Units are units in general hospitals, sometimes only a ward. They offer mainly short-term treatment. Psychiatric Hospitals are small compared with the Public Mental Hospitals and provide largely short-term treatment. Hospitals for Addicts are in-patient facilities for both alcoholics and drug addicts.

This table tells us that women's overall share of the total who were admitted for the first time to a psychiatric facility in Canada in 1970 was 48 per cent, slightly less than half. The overall figure however conceals rather wide variations. The percentage of women in Federal Psychiatric Units is very small – only 0.3%. *Statistics Canada* doesn't tell us exactly what Federal Psychiatric Units are, but most probably they are in some way comparable to the Veterans Administration facilities in the U.S. in drawing from a largely male population, either in the Canadian armed forces or possibly from federal penitentiaries (in any case the overall numbers are rather small – only 728).

Public Mental Hospitals and Psychiatric Units in general hospitals provide for about three-quarters (76%) of all first admissions to in-patient treatment. These two seem complementary. Women are only 39% of first admissions to public mental hospitals, but are 60% of admissions to private psychiatric units. They are slightly less than half (47% of first admissions) to Psychiatric Units and have a relatively small share of first admissions to Hospitals for Addicts (only 21%).

One thing *Statistics Canada* enables us to check out is how the kinds of numbers we are trying to interpret might be affected by different numbers of women and men in the population.

TABLE 2

All institutions, first admissions by sex and age (ages 15-59), all diagnostic categories, (rates per 100,000 population).

	15-19	20-29	30-39	40-49	50-59
Women	300	344	373	329	261
Men	298	356	369	393	317

Note: This table does not exclude organic mental illnesses, senile dementias and diseases of childhood. I used the *Statistics Canada* material directly since the information needed to recalculate the rates was not readily available.

In Table 2 we can look at differences in first admissions for women and men of different ages in proportion to the numbers of women and men in the population at each of those ages.

Out of every hundred thousand women between 15 and 19 living in Canada in 1970, 300 were admitted to a public psychiatric facility of some kind. The rate for men of that age is about the same. Between the ages of 20 and 29, 344 women out of every hundred thousand were admitted for the first time to a public psychiatric facility. The rate for men in that age group is somewhat higher — 356 in every hundred thousand. *In only one age group are the rates for women significantly higher than the rates for men.* This is the age group 30-39. Out of every hundred thousand women between those ages living in Canada in 1970, 373 were hospitalized for the first time as mentally ill. The rate for men at that age is a little lower, only 369 out of every hundred thousand. At later ages however the rates for men exceed those for women.

The figures that we've looked at so far don't give us quite the same picture as Chesler's. As compared with men, we don't find a consistently large female involvement. Only one type of facility, Public Psychiatric Units, show proportionately more women than men. These would probably be comparable to the general psychiatric wards in Chesler's figures. The public mental hospitals are roughly comparable to state and county hospitals in the U.S. and here the Canadian figures show a predominance of men, as compared to apparently equal numbers of men and women in the States. Overall the Canadian figures show slightly lower proportions of women than men in residential facilities. Is this because we're looking at a different society with different problems for women and for men? They certainly don't show women experiencing more mental illness than men. If anything the opposite. Or are there problems in how Chesler has presented the state of affairs in the U.S.? Has she in fact described it properly?

Here are some reasons for the difference in what the official Canadian and U.S. figures say

1. The picture could be different because the statistics used are put together differently. For example, Chesler is using numbers of people 'in treatment' whereas *Statistics Canada* gives us 'first admissions.' People institutionalized during any one year include people who may be admitted for the second or third time. First admissions, on the other hand, tell you only the people who are being admitted for the first time. This

can give you for any year an idea of how many people are becoming mentally ill but it doesn't tell you how many people are in treatment come the time the institution makes up its books. Obviously there could be a difference here. Chesler suggests that women are more likely to stay and more likely to be readmitted.[5] If this is so, similar figures for women and men on first admissions would show up as more women than men on the institutional books at book-keeping time.

2. I've cut the cake differently because I have left out the over-60s. For over-60s you must compare rates rather than, as Chesler does, the overall numbers. We don't know from Chesler's data how far the differences she finds between women and men result from factors of this sort. We can't take for granted as we can for the ages between 15-59 that the numbers of men and women at all ages are more or less the same. We know that women tend to live longer than men, and that there are therefore more women than men in the over-60 group. There are likely to be more women in treatment in this age group simply because there are more women than men in it. We can't wash out this possibility without comparing the rates. (If you want to see the difference made by comparing *rates* as against comparing numbers and proportions, check Table A in the appendix showing the numbers of women and men and the percentage of women admitted at various ages against Table 2 above showing the rates per 100,000 population.)

3. Perhaps Chesler's descriptions focus on figures which show more mental illness among women than men and neglect those that don't show this or show the opposite.

Her account of the increase in numbers of women overall and relative to men from 1964 to 1968 sounds pretty impressive in absolute numbers. But if we compare the shares women and men have in a total figure which increases year by year, then the increase of women over men becomes much less dramatic — over the five year period women's share has increased by only 2 percentage points from 50% to 52%. (Table 3)

4. Along the same lines in her description of the difference in percentages of women and men in treatment, she doesn't mention the much greater numbers of men in Veterans Administration hospitals and out-patient services. In 1968 there were 61,493 men in VA in- and out-patient care and only 2,220 women. Women of course are less likely to have been in the

armed services and thus less likely to be entitled to use VA facilities. Why doesn't Chesler include them in her discussion (they are included in her overall figures)? Perhaps because this explanation for a difference between the sexes doesn't fit into the framework she (and we) are working with. It tells us something about administrative practices of the U.S. government. It doesn't tell us anything about how social contexts may cause emotional disturbance. So it gets left out. But since much mental illness among men is being treated in these facilities, that omission introduces a bias into the discussion.

Perhaps after all there isn't much difference between the Canadian figures and the U.S. ones. Certainly Chesler's formidable description is beginning to seem much less well grounded. The differences which seem so clear and strong on first reading become ambiguous when we look at them closely.

TABLE 3

Chesler recalculated (from her Table 4, *Women and Madness*, p. 313). Women as percentage of total population by each of six psychiatric facilities, (U.S.) 1964-1968 inclusive.

	Women as % of total	Totals (100%)
1964	50 (479,167)	957,255
1965	50 (543,738)	1,077,843
1966	51 (538,682)	1,055,351
1967	52 (594,225)	1,147,827
1968	52 (615,122)	1,179,861

Note: Numbers are in brackets after percentages.

Another American study done by Gove & Tudor [6] comes up with findings similar to Chesler's but based on different types of statistical information. They believe that women's role in modern industrial societies has characteristics which are likely to produce higher rates of mental illness among women than men. They bring together a lot of information including studies which have been done on the use of out-patient facilities. They conclude

> The information on first admissions to mental hospitals, psychiatric treatment in general hospitals, psychiatric out-patient clinics, private out-patient care, the practices of general physicians, and community surveys all indicate that more women than men are mentally ill.[7]

Of course they are using some information from sources we do not have (from private out-patient care, practices of general physicians and community surveys – and it is a very useful study in bringing together a lot of material). But they are using first admissions and so far as their information overlaps with the statistics we've looked at already, the Canadian figures don't show that more women than men are mentally ill. On the basis of these figures, their generalizations aren't confirmed for Canada. If anything, the opposite. Why this difference?

Gove & Tudor treat mental illness in a special way. They define it so as to exclude some of the kinds of problems which bring people into psychiatric treatment or care, and which therefore get counted in the overall figures. Mental illness is a very loose category which covers almost anything that can turn up in treatment or care in a psychiatric agency. Gove & Tudor refine it and narrow it down so that the term applies to a single range of problems only. In their view mental illness is

> a disorder which involves personal discomfort (as indicated by distress, anxiety, etc.) and/or mental disorganization (as indicated by confusion, thought blockage, motor retardation, and, in the more extreme cases, by hallucinations and delusions) that is not caused by an organic or toxic condition.[8]

Gove and Tudor have defined mental illness in terms of states of feeling, or emotion, and mental states. In their view it is a disorder of mental or emotional processes which is not part of an organic disease and doesn't result from using drugs or alcohol.

When patients are admitted to psychiatric facilities of the kind we are concerned with here, they are given a diagnosis. The system of diagnosis used in the U.S. and Canada is more or less the same. Some diagnostic categories fit with their definition and others don't. In looking for evidence in the kinds of

 statistical materials we've used here Gove & Tudor focus on

four diagnostic categories, two major – these are the neurotic disorders and functional psychoses, and two minor – transient situational disorders and somatic disorders of psychic origin. Relatively very few are diagnosed in the last category and for the purposes of our discussion, I'm going to leave it out.

Neurotic disorder is defined by Gove & Tudor as "anxiety in the absence of psychotic disorganization."[9] The difference between neurosis and psychosis is mainly that in the latter there are problems with processes of thinking or with how the patient perceives and understands what is happening, whereas neuroses are mainly emotional difficulties.

Gove & Tudor exclude, as we have, all forms of mental illness arising from organic causes. They also apparently exclude mental illness originating in or identified with 'toxic' conditions such as alcoholism. They also exclude a diagnostic category called 'personality disorders.' They do so because, they argue, people identified in this way are non-conforming in ways which are disruptive to others, but they don't themselves experience mental distress. Therefore they don't fit their definition of mental illness.

This all makes perfectly good sense. It is by proceeding on this basis that they are able to come up with the conclusion that more women than men are mentally ill. This is a conclusion that *applies to this meaning of mental illness only* and *does not apply* to mental illness as it's generally and casually used by all of us to talk about almost anything that gets you into a psychiatric facility as an in-patient.

There is a problem however. It is this. When we look at how women and men are distributed in the various diagnostic categories in the Canadian figures, we find a quite definite pattern with some of them. It is described as follows by *Statistics Canada*:

> Mental disorders such as alcoholism, alcoholic psychosis, personality disorders, sexual deviations, and drug dependence continued to be predominantly male disorders, while neuroses and affective psychoses continued to be predominantly female disorders.[10]

The way in which Gove & Tudor have defined mental illness excludes from consideration at the outset all those types of disorder in which men predominate – at least in the Canadian figures. Here is how this works. What I've done is to take a table which you'll find at the end of this paper (Table B in the appendix) and put it together in Gove & Tudor terms. I have left out sexual deviations because Gove & Tudor do (and because, as you can see for yourself, the numbers are extremely small) and also for obvious reasons 'other and unspecified.' Alcoholism and alcoholic psychoses and drug dependence are excluded by the rule which excludes conditions caused by toxins (they may also be excluded by how administrative responsibilities are defined). We have already seen how personality disorders were excluded.

TABLE 4

Gove & Tudor's definition of mental illness is used to analyze the data on mental disorders focussing on those described by *Statistics Canada* as predominantly female or male.

Mental illness according to Gove & Tudor

	Women as % of total	Total 100%
Functional psychoses - total	52 (4,760)	9,077
Schizophrenia	46 (2,503)	5,403
Affective psychosis	63 (1,966)	3,113
Paranoid states	52 (291)	561
Neuroses	64 (8,945)	13,931
Transient Situational disturbance	58 (1,011)	1,742
Gove & Tudor mental illness total	59 (14,716)	24,750

Not mental illness according to Gove & Tudor

	Women as % of total	Total 100%
Personality disorders	41 (1,417)	3,466
Alcoholism & Alcoholic psychoses	15 (1,147)	7,590
Drug dependence	32 (393)	1,241
Gove & Tudor non-mental illness - total	24 (2,957)	12,297
Overall Total	48 (17,673)	37,047

Note 1: The numbers of women appear in brackets after the percentages.
Note 2: This table is based on the information contained in Table B in the appendix.

This table lays a Gove & Tudor grid over the *Statistics Canada* data. When we look at the diagnostic categories defined by Gove & Tudor as mental illness, that is, the functional psychoses with their sub-categories of schizophrenia, affective psychoses (major emotional disorders such as depressions, manic states, etc.), and paranoid states, and the neuroses and transient situational disturbances women clearly have a larger share of the total than men. The overall figure is 59%. Within the category of functional psychoses there is some variation – somewhat more men than women are diagnosed as schizophrenic and the difference between women and men for the category for functional psychoses as a whole is relatively insignificant (52%women). The major disproportions between women and men are found in the sub-category of functional psychoses, affective psychoses and neuroses. Women are 63% of those diagnosed as suffering from affective psychoses on first admission and 64% of those diagnosed as suffering from neuroses.

If we pick up however on the *Statistics Canada* picture and add in those kinds of disorders which are not clearly part of an organic disease, we find that it is here that men predominate. Gove & Tudor exclude Alcoholic Psychoses and Alcoholism and Drug Dependence by their rule excluding conditions caused by toxins. Yet women's share of the total diagnosed as some form of alcoholic problem is only 15% and is only 32% of the total diagnosed as suffering from drug dependence on their first admission to in-patient treatment. Gove & Tudor define personality disorders out of the picture and here again women's share of the total is noticeably less than men's – only 41%. Combining all these three diagnostic categories we find that women are only 24% of the total as compared with 60% of Gove & Tudor type mental illness.[12]

We can see the pattern identified by *Statistics Canada* quite clearly. When we lay the Gove & Tudor definition of mental illness like a grid over the *Statistics Canada* figures, what we find is troublesome. It suggests that Gove & Tudor have selected a definition which eliminates all the diagnostic categories in which men predominate over women, with the exception of schizophrenia where the difference is not great. Certainly this is how it works when we apply it to the Canadian figures. If we accept the Gove & Tudor definition, women in Canada do have a markedly larger share of the total who are admitted to psychiatric facilities as mentally ill. There are 60% women in this category and only 40% men – a 20 percentage points difference. But when we include those that Gove & Tudor exclude, this difference disappears. In fact women with 48% have a slightly lower share of that total than men, with 52%.

If we think about it further, their reasons for ruling out the diagnostic categories in which men predominate seem thin. Alcoholism doesn't originate in a toxic condition and nor does Drug Dependence. Might not their criterion of experienced mental distress rule out some people diagnosed as schizophrenic, as suffering from affective psychoses (manic type) and some neuroses? We must in any case be suspicious of so neat an outcome as this.

In arguing with Chesler and Gove & Tudor, we've begun to find out something about the picture provided by the official Canadian statistics. These show us that the shares of women and men in the over-all numbers first admitted to treatment in various psychiatric agencies named are about equal. If anything rather fewer women than men come into treatment or care. But the overall figures hide some pretty wide variations. The main ones are these:

1. Different kinds of agencies seem to some degree to specialize in one sex or the other. More men than women are admitted for the first time to Public Mental Hospitals and Hospitals for Addicts. On the other hand more women than men are admitted to Public Psychiatric Units (see Table 1). Both Chesler and Gove & Tudor report studies showing that women have a bigger share than men in the use of psychiatric out-patient facilities. That's something we haven't looked at yet, but we will return to it when we have a second look at the statistics in the last section of the paper.

2. Rates of mental illness also vary with age, and women and men differ here also. For most ages according to the Canadian statistics, fewer women than men in proportion to their numbers in the population at that age are admitted to one of the named psychiatric agencies. There is one age group in which the rates for women are higher than for men. Between the ages of 30-39, 373 women in every 100,000 women in Canada between those ages are admitted as compared with 369 men per 100,000 population (Table 2).

3. Finally, when we looked at the Gove & Tudor information in relation to what we found in *Statistics Canada*, another source of variation concealed by the overall figures emerged. There are what *Statistics Canada* call "female and male disorders." This means simply that women predominate markedly over men in some types of psychiatric diagnosis (notably in Affective Psychoses and to a lesser extent in Paranoid States) whereas men predominate (very markedly) in the

diagnostic categories of Alcoholism, Drug Dependence and Personality Disorders.

What we'd like to be able to do with the Canadian statistics is pretty much what Chesler and Gove & Tudor have done. We'd like to be able to read back through the statistical information to actual states of mental illness which can be related to the oppression women experience in contemporary society. But when we try to do this we run into difficulties. The points we have criticized in how Chesler and Gove & Tudor have interpreted the information available are problems which people working in this area and trying to do just this kind of thing run into again and again. People have had to make do with the official statistical information or with statistical data specifically created for the purpose. In both cases, special kinds of operations have to be done on the data to strip it down and purify it so that somehow it will speak only of mental illness and can be treated as representing where mental illness is located and how distributed in a given population. This always involves the ditching of some kind of administrative or professional detritus which seems an arbitrary source of variation in the data (i.e., one which doesn't have anything to do with the main focus upon mental illness as a state of the individual existing independently of how psychiatric agencies work). Chesler, for example, dumps the Veterans Administration figures in her discussion.[13] Here the bias towards men is *clearly administrative*. Those figures don't lend themselves to an interpretation which is interested in being able to go from numbers of women versus men in psychiatric agencies to the social causes of the differences. Gove & Tudor adopt a special strategy. They clean up the idea of mental illness so that it simply omits the diagnostic categories in which men predominate (Alcoholism, Drug Dependence and Personality Disorders) – at least according to *Statistics Canada*.

Each clean-up job makes perfectly good sense on its own, but each next time a clean-up job is done – each time *something* has to be left out or not said in order to make it possible to read from the statistics to actual states of mental illness in a population – we must ask whether any one of them or any new one we could think of would do the job. These problems crop up again and again in studying mental illness. Perhaps there's no way the statistical information can be decontaminated.

III
Ways of thinking about mental illness

I'd like to introduce an alternative. It is that we don't try to clean up the statistical information. Throwing out this or that in order to penetrate to the *real thing* which we suppose to be out there in back of them implies a particular way of thinking about mental illness. This assumes that it is a state of the individual which can be separated from what is happening to her in the psychiatric context. A number of recent thinkers in this field have argued that becoming mentally ill is a process in which psychiatric agencies participate. Put simply in terms of the statistical information - this means that when you seem to be counting people becoming mentally ill you are in fact also counting what psychiatric agencies do. The two aspects can't be taken apart. *The figures can't be decontaminated.*

In interpreting any kind of factual information, we have to use some kind of method of thinking which shapes what is there into categories of objects and decides what kinds of connections we are going to make between them. Gove & Tudor use a very general method. Chesler's approach is harder to pin down, but belongs to the same general type.[14] I'm going to describe it in very simplified terms. And then using the work of Szasz (1961),[15] Scheff (1962)[16] and Laing [17] I'm going to suggest an alternative method of thinking about mental illness.

The method of thinking that requires us to clean up the data begins with mental illness as a distinct state of the individual which is recognizable in symptoms. You can tell when this state exists and its nature by examining, by observing or being told about the individual's symptoms. The symptoms are definite types of behaviour which can be identified and named. This state may have various causes. One type of cause is believed to be social situations which cause stress. In such situations and over a period of time individuals experiencing stress may become emotionally disturbed. As the underlying state of mental illness develops it becomes observable to herself or others as symptoms. At some point she or her relatives or friends put her in touch with a psychiatric agency. Her illness is diagnosed and she is counted (thereby producing the statistical information through which we can reach back to the original state of mental illness). Briefly it goes like this: there is first a situation which causes stress. This leads to mental illness. The mental illness is treated professionally – hence the statistical information. As it is generally used, this method of thinking about mental illness can be diagrammed thus:

Figure 1.

stages:

1		2		3		4
oppressive social situation	**→**	**stress**	**→**	**mental illness**	**→**	**control by psychiatric agency**

To bring it round to where we are, we could add a stage 5, the statistics. The different stages are distinct. The connections represented by the arrows are simple (causal type) connections and they all go in the same direction. It is this method of thinking which makes it possible to begin with statistical information created at stage 4 and use it to learn about relations between stages 1 and 3. The key 'elements' – social situation, mental illness and psychiatric agency are all distinct and fully separated from one another. Mental illness is out there as a distinct state. It comes into being *before* an individual goes for treatment. It may be *caused* by social situations but it is *separable* from them. There may be some slippage between becoming mentally ill and going for treatment because of such things as lack of facilities, inadequate knowledge about mental illness, prejudice, and etc. There may be inadequacies in the book-keeping procedures used by psychiatric agencies. But there is no doubt that in principle you can, just as with other diseases, go from the book-keeping procedures of the treatment agency to talking about distribution of the problem in the population. That's what is generally attempted. It's because this model is used that cleaning up things which muddle the clarity of the connections (the general practice) or cleaning up the thing itself (as Gove & Tudor do with the category of mental illness) make sense.

The alternative says that mental illness can't be separated as a thing, object, state, disease entity (or what have you) from the social operations of psychiatry. Szasz [18] and Scheff [19] have suggested that there is no such thing as mental illness; that there is nothing at all which the statistics point back to which is a definite entity.

Szasz' view is that people come to psychiatric agencies for many kinds of problems. People experience despair and misery. There are many forms of suffering and of psychological malfunctioning of various depths and degrees. Most of these, in his view, arise out of facets of the human social condition. They are packaged as mental illness by the psychiatric agencies.

These agencies sort them out, put them in categories, work their technical work upon them, and/or shut people up in places apart. The mentally ill are the people upon whom this work is done. And that is all they have in common.[20]

Scheff takes a rather similar view. He suggests that becoming mentally ill begins with various and vague ways in which people's behaviour doesn't fit with what other people see as standard ways of doing things. Mental illness is rather like the file marked miscellaneous. After all the other ways in which people break rules have been named, identified and dealt with by their appropriate agencies of control (the law courts, the schools for the handicapped, etc., etc.) there is a bundle left over which doesn't fit any one of these. He calls these *residual* deviations. Most people deviate in these ways. Sometimes these deviations lead to psychiatric treatment. When this happens, that individual begins to play the role of being mentally ill. What we call symptoms are behaviour appropriate to the role which people have learned to play in the psychiatric context.[21]

A fundamental problem is that unless you are concerned with a kind of mental illness that has a definite physical basis, objective criteria for recognizing behaviour as the symptoms of mental illness or otherwise establishing that someone is mentally ill are hard to come by. Mental illness is not out there to be observed like a rock or a buttercup or a planet or even like measles. Nor as Scheff[22] points out is there any definite rule or set of rules which people who are identified as mentally ill can be said to have broken or deviated from.

Seeing what people do as symptoms of mental illness is something that comes about between people in interaction with one another. Symptoms are not observable independently of actual settings in which people are relating to one another. There are always two parties to a symptom. We generally don't pay attention to this when one of them is a professional whose position is theoretically one of detachment. He is examining the patient. The patient is there behaving for him to examine. And so on. But being detached is a special way of relating to people. Examining someone is a special kind of interaction.[23] Therefore it isn't clear how the behaviour of people described as mentally ill can be considered as 'wrong' in a way which separates that judgment from particular individuals (relatives, friends, psychiatrists, psychologists, and others) encountering particular people (a friend, a child, a wife, a husband, a patient) in particular settings (at home, in a psychiatrist's office, in a hospital ward, etc.).

There have been many attempts to locate mental illness in the community before people have made contact with a psychiatric agency. Interview methods rather than the official statistics of admissions, etc. have been used. But these also are subject to this more general difficulty — that the judgment of whether anything is wrong or what is wrong is always made by people who begin with particular understandings of behaviour and with particular ideas about mental illness. These kinds of background understandings are built into how we see others. We can't escape that. They are essentially part of *any* relationship, *any* conversation, *any* interaction, *any* understanding of behaviour. Each person brings to a situation her understanding of what is going on . What happens there is partly a product of how she understood it.

This means also that psychiatric diagnoses are not like the diagnoses of disease which depend upon physical symptoms or signs. It is the functioning of the individual in routine situations which becomes the problem. How she behaves depends on the situation, on others present and how they interpret what she does. Knowing who she is, that she is a she, that she comes from this or that kind of background, that her age is thus and so — these considerations enter into the picture that leads to the diagnosis. The psychiatrist already works with an array of typical pictures of the kind of person who is schizophrenic, who is neurotic, who is alcoholic, etc.

The types include characterizations of sex and age. They include notions of the behaviour appropriate for women and for men. They include judgments about people's physical appearance. And so on and so on. Diagnoses and dispositional decisions (decisions about where to place someone) and decisions about treatment include this *invisible* judgmental work on the part of psychiatric professionals. This same work thus also counts in the book-keeping operations of psychiatric agencies.

Furthermore, one major dimension of interpretation which enters into the relation of everyone towards someone who has been defined as mentally ill is just that. Once someone has been labelled mentally ill, they are related to in those terms. They are not expected to make sense so people tend not to listen to or respond to them as if they do.

The attitude can be summarized as a set of instructions which tell us how to respond to someone who "is" mentally ill. The first instruction says something like "Find out how to see this person's behaviour as not making sense."[24] One method of doing this is to separate the person's behaviour from the situations in which it belongs. This is done routinely in psychiatric settings, both by the way in which the patient is seen outside her lived settings and by the way in which the psychiatric procedures of making accounts and clinical description lift pieces of behaviour out of context (as we'll see in an example given in the next section – IV). In any case if your instructions tell you to make nonsense of what people do, it's surprisingly easy to do it. The second set of instructions might say something like "Don't relate to this person as if you could look at the world from the same place." People don't relate to people who "are" mentally ill in the same way as they relate to others. They don't readily enter into a "we" relation with them in which it is taken for granted that both share the same space, the same social and temporal coordinates and experience things from the base of a shared set of conditions. And finally, there's a third set of instructions saying something like "Don't take what she says seriously. Don't make it into anything which counts for you as something to act upon or respond to." This is something like a "don't trust her" kind of instruction but it goes further than that because it means that what she says and does is discredited or discounted as a basis for action. For example, if she who has been labelled mentally ill is angry with you, this instruction tells you not to treat that anger as a reason for getting angry back or asking yourself what you've done or the like.

These instructions seal off people labelled as mentally ill from ordinary social participation. The experience of people who are unimpeachably normal going unrecognized as such in a mental hospital is the work of what I've represented as this set of instructions.[25]

Whatever it is that gets called mental illness becomes recognizably and distinctly what it is for the official record, in psychiatric offices, admissions suites of mental hospitals, the intake practices of clinics and etc. It is a whole relation to the world which the person becoming mentally ill in this sense discovers. When she is being put on record she is already in a relation to the world which is changed for her. This is the relation of mental illness. There is no phenomena of mental illness which can be separated from the same procedures which produces the statistics. The agencies which produce the statistics also produce mental illness. They don't produce the suffering, the despair, the misery, the loss of self which leads in one way or another to someone's *entry* to the psychiatric process, but they do produce the distinctive behaviours, how they are recorded and understood and that pattern of relating to others *which we call mental illness*.

This doesn't mean that what is happening to individuals which leads them into contact with psychiatry is not real. We have to understand that there are experiences which are overwhelmingly fearful, states of total suspension in diffuse anxiety, conditions of profound despair and grief; and further that in relation to others, there are also times and people with whom others cannot live, or who make others afraid for themselves (we see here again how troubles are defined interactionally). We begin to call others – or ourselves – mentally ill as a way of organizing these kinds of responses leading up to doing something of a very definite kind about them.

All this means that we can't go back through the statistics to find either a definite phenomenon which we can call mental illness, or a way of counting it which ensures that we are counting *something* and something we can properly treat as being the same sort of thing (allowing for errors) every time we count it. Nor can we separate what is called mental illness from what we'd like to view as its cause. Nor can we separate the processes by which people come to be counted as mentally ill (by coming into treatment usually) from the ways in which being under the psychiatric jurisdiction changes how others relate to them. This changes both how they relate *and* how they are seen to relate, responded to, and interpreted. To be there (and that happened to me) and under that kind of scrutiny, changes all your relations to the world and to yourself. That special experience can't be separated from the experience of being or becoming mentally ill and can't be separated from the behaviour and responses which lead to people being labelled as mentally ill. (Let alone the sometimes radically stressful and frightening experiences which some experience in mental hospitals.)

We could rewrite our model for thinking about mental illness like this

Figure 2.

1	2	3	4
oppressive social situation →	**stress →**	**psychiatric control →**	**mental illness**

Most people thinking along these lines don't view mental illness as actually *caused* by psychiatric intervention, but rather take the view that wherever it originates it takes on its particular character in the social contexts created by psychiatry. It *becomes* mental illness – rather than something else – in that context. (And that has consequences then for what *she* becomes.)

IV
Cleaning up

We must drop the idea that we can track back through the statistics on mental illness to find out about a reality hidden behind them which they represent. They are figures which are not put together to draw a representation. We can't reach in back of them or through them as if they were a dirty glass through which we could have a perfect picture if we could only clean it up. *Statistics Canada* in their introduction to their statistical information, tell us that we have to be careful in reading and interpreting their data. This is what they say:

> The level and rate of change of first admissions by province should be interpreted against a backdrop of existing services for the mentally ill, the number of psychiatric beds available; the official and unofficial admission policies of the psychiatric facilities; the extent of health insurance coverage for the various mental disorders; demographic characteristics such as the population size, and composition by age and marital status; sociological factors such as the degree of urbanization, and attitudes toward psychiatric facilities and the mentally ill. Each province incorporates a unique constellation of these factors which determine the extent of provincial variations in psychiatric inpatient movement.[26]

An alternative to these precautionary measures and to the kind of interpretation we have been criticizing is to turn the problem on its head. How is it that these varieties of relations between psychiatric facilities and community can produce a coherent and *apparently* unproblematic collection of statistical information? How does all this mess get cleaned up so that it can be presented as it is and used as it does so often get used? I think we have to think about the figures differently and in fact much more straightforwardly. We have to begin by asking questions about how they are produced. How do they come about as we find them on the books? What are the institutional processes which produce them? What sorts of work contexts among professionals and others are the contexts in which the routine work of producing the data to be counted gets done? How are these varieties of experience, situation, policy, practice, conditions and exigencies worked up into the forms in which they are made thus simply accountable? If we focus on *this* as the 'reality' which lies in back of the statistical information, perhaps we can begin to say something about it in a rather different way. Thus the question this section attempts to answer is: How are these *standardized and general* forms of statistical information produced out of the *varieties of particular local contexts* which *Statistics Canada* describes? I am going to present a general picture of the processes involved in getting this done.[27]

We begin with the observation (obvious but usually neglected) that the statistics on mental illness are put together as part of a system of professional and bureaucratic book-keeping. Governments are necessarily interested in such things as the costs of psychiatric services and the 'needs' of the population. They are concerned with how many people come into treatment, how many are in care during particular accounting periods, what types of facilities are being used and by whom, and what are the alternative sources of support (family, lack of family, etc.). Their interests in the statistics are different from ours and from those of researchers into the 'causes' of mental illness. We make second-hand use of information which is collected for other purposes.

Further, the character of the statistical information is shaped by the role these reports have traditionally played in the system of governmental control over psychiatric facilities. For example, the statistics on mental hospitalization that are to be found in earlier Annual Reports of the Mental Health Branch of the British Columbia Department of Health give information organized exclusively round the economics of running mental hospitals. Their books on patients show only admissions, discharges, deaths, etc. Until 1972 they gave no information about the age or sex of patients. They just counted how many came in, how many were on the books and how many left either by discharge or death. *Statistics Canada* Mental Health information appears to have been elaborated from a similar base – the ordinary operation of in-patient psychiatric facilities. Various additional pieces of information have been added on. Diagnostic categories, and the marital status of patients as well as their age and sex, are included.

There is however no information about the occupational, educational or income levels of patients or where they came from. (Anything that would allow the reader to tie down some of the factors mentioned by *Statistics Canada* in their preliminary warning is lacking.)

The production of such statistical information is part of an extensive bureaucratic and professional organization. It includes of course the work of transforming the raw material of the world into the forms in which they can be processed as data. This work gets done almost invisibly as part of the routine work and routine use of skill by psychiatric professionals. Psychiatrists, psychologists, social workers and psychiatric nurses learn their specialized roles in training institutions which are part of a national and in most instances an international professional structure. The ways in which psychiatric care is organized and how patients are talked about, treated and categorized are standardized in this training process. Using the textbooks, journals, and other media of their profession, they learn to think psychiatrically, to talk psychiatrically, to describe what is happening in the terms of their discipline, and to recognize and name patient's problems properly. They learn thus to produce the kinds of accounts that go into the work of psychiatric book-keeping and they learn, of course, to construct the kinds of accounts of people implied by the psychiatric and psychological ideologies described elsewhere in this book by Kimball,[28] King,[29] and Smith.[30]

As part of the same process they learn how to go about relating to people in the kinds of situations they will encounter them in – the various settings of ward and office, of coffee room and hallway, of lecture theatre and convention hotel, which are the typical occasions of psychiatric encounter. They learn how to relate to members of their own professions and to those of others and they learn how to talk to patients, how to talk about patients and how to talk *to* patients so as to be able to talk *about* patients.

The bureaucratic and professional terminologies and methods of making accounts of these various (and more or less formal kinds) are not inessential. They cannot be arbitrarily dispensed with. The terms and methods of accounting for and describing what is being done set the forms under which people recognize what they do and what others do as properly actionable. Errington [31], in a study of the workings of a police phone room, has shown how the kinds of problems callers telephone in with are shaped up in the police response on the phone into the forms which fit the various possible 'bureaucratic' responses – including of course the response of doing nothing. The world that people live in and in which their troubles arise is "entered" into the systems set up to control it by fitting them and their troubles to standardized terms and procedures under which they can be formally recognized and made actionable. These processes are *intrinsic* to the workings of professional and bureaucratic forms of organization. They are *essential* to the making and implementing of policies, including policies about what kinds of patients shall be admitted to a facility and therefore what kinds of numbers and statuses (marital status, age, etc.) will turn up in the final and simplified accountings of the government statistics.

Professional and bureaucratic procedures and terminologies are part of an abstracted system. Abstracted systems are set up to be independent of the particular, the individual, the idiosyncratic and the local. Hence the specialized forms of training referred to above. Hence also the continual processes of working up and maintaining the standard sets of terms, procedures, etc. which are part of the work done in conferences, journals, and other forms of professional communication. In actual operation however *the abstracted forms must be fitted to the actual local situations* in which they must function and which they control. In practice the abstracted system has to be tied into the local and particular. Psychiatric agencies have to develop ways of working which fit situations and people who are not standardized, don't present standardized problems, and are not already shaped up into the forms under which they can be recognized in the terms which make them actionable. What actually happens, what people actually do and experience, the real situations they function in, how they get to agencies – none of these things is neatly shaped up. There is a process of practical interchange between an inexhaustibly messy and different and indefinite real world and the bureaucratic and professional system which controls and acts upon it. The professional is trained to produce out of this the order which he believes he discovers in it.

Psychiatric agencies articulate the bureaucratic and professional structures to the local setting. The application of psychiatric methods of making accounts gets worked out in the actual situations which arise in the community. Local conditions and troubles characteristic of them – the isolation of the housewife living in a trailer in a northern company town; the psychic and physical exhaustion of women overborn by caring for children under conditions of poverty; the man who keeps himself going at the pulp mill by drinking himself blind every night; the young man whose efforts at autonomy from his family are treated as sickness – recurrent social situations create typical local uses for psychiatric facilities. An interface of routine operating develops which transposes these recurrent and characteristic local uses into the psychiatric and administrative terms which make them actionable.

Different kinds of psychiatric agencies are set up with different capabilities and more or less specialized services. The latter are built into staffing patterns, types of premises, budgets, locations, etc. As agencies become articulated to the local community their capabilities and services become part of a social organization which settles what their actual uses will be, the kinds of problems which reach them, what we might describe as their administrative constituency (how agencies such as police, welfare, etc. use them) and their clientele. The uses of available agencies is the outcome of what the agency offers, the kinds of problems emerging in the community which it can handle and the fit that is created between the two by the social connections of referral, health insurance, welfare, police practice, word-of-mouth and etc. The transposition of what happens and is happening to people where their problems originate into recognizable psychiatric forms is done in part by the social organization which connects agency and patient. There is a process of working up which is not done by any particular individual but is a concerted action in which agencies such as welfare, the police, the patient herself or her relatives are involved before she ever gets to the psychiatric facility. Further work is done by the various personnel of the agency, receptionists, social workers, nurses, as well as psychiatrists. Events and people get shaped up in a whole variety of ways by routinely standardizing the settings in which they are observed, by asking them and others standardized questions, by isolating them from their personal and idiosyncratic situations, by controlling what they can say and how it is listened to, and so on. Much of what is really part of their lives and their experience simply disappears in this process. It ceases to be visible. How they came to the agency isn't visible except as perhaps a brief formality. The kinds of uses they or others are making of the agency also disappear.

People working professionally in psychiatric agencies and similar organizations come to experience people's problems as types in relation to the kinds of actions to be taken. Types are an integral part of the process which fits the abstracted terms of the profession or bureaucracy to the actual situations.[32] They work as a matching process which assembles, selects and organizes within a specialized context. The individual is already distant from her biography and her lived situation. She is encountered and experienced as patient in the special settings of office, ward, foyer of hospital, interview room or the like. She is encountered in the form of a case history already written and through the forms of interview which disclose only the pieces of her life which fall into the slots. She is encountered also in the context of the routine performance of professional work, as part of what the psychiatrist (or other professional) has to get through with that day. The experiences which are recurrent for the psychiatrist and which he has learned to name and describe as types of patients result from the characteristic local 'uses' of the agency but do not include them.

The clinical entities of mental illness are formal descriptions of types originating in clinical experience and included in authoritative textbooks and similar sources. They provide for psychiatrists (and others) a template to which the patterning of their experience is to be fitted. Here are two passages from autobiographies describing experiences which could be but have not been, fitted to such a template. They are followed by a third passage from a clinical description which shows the template to which they could be matched. This process of matching which you do yourself *is* the process I am describing.

Here is the first. Margery Spring Rice in a book called *Working Class Wives*, published in 1939 and reflecting the depression years in England, gives this account by a working class woman.

> This constant struggle with poverty this last four years has made me feel very nervy and irritable and this affects my children. I fear I have not the patience that good health generally brings. When I am especially worried about anything I feel as if I have been engaged in some terrific physical struggle and go utterly limp and for some time am unable to move or even think coherently. This effect of mental strain expressed in physical results seems most curious and I am at a loss to properly explain it to a doctor.[33]

This is an account of subjective experience – insider's knowledge. Here is a description by an outside observer of what could be the same experience. Ms. Knight in her autobiography *A Very Ordinary Life* [34] describes how hard her mother had to work and how little help she got from her husband (the time is early 20th century and the place Germany).

> We children didn't realize how badly he was treating our mother then. Sometimes we would find her sitting in a corner staring vacantly across the room...She used to sit behind the door sometimes, in a space between the wall and a large wardrobe. There she would sit, still and staring. We kids would open the door quietly and peep in. "Is Mama still sitting there?" "Yes, still there." No supper, no light, nothing. She'd sit there for hours sometimes.[35]

In taking these excerpts I have isolated them from context. This is particularly marked in the second where I can see that by picking out what is psychiatrically describable (by the clinical description of depression which follows) I have already changed the character of the description by changing its relation to its setting. I *aimed* at making it describable in some such way. Ms. Knight's mother already looks sicker than she does when you see the full record of what she contended with and how effectively she did so.

Here is a psychiatrist's description of 'depressive illness.' I have chosen one written for lay persons so as to avoid technical language. And I have chosen one which *could* describe both the foregoing examples. The essentials of the typing procedures involved in making clinical descriptions are visible.[36] According to Sir David Stafford-Clark, the illness of depression is characterized by

> some blunting and withdrawal of interest from the outside world, a general slowing up of mental and physical activity so that the patient thinks and responds to questions only with difficulty and after a struggle, and may even display a hesitation and retardation in movement as well as in thought...
>
> In some cases (inertia and retardation of response) may go on into a condition of complete stupor wherein the patient sits or lies motionless and unresponsive, completely aware of what is going on around him but no longer able or disposed to do anything about it.[37]

 As I've said, this passage could describe both the other two. In it we can see how they might look made over into a clinical description. They would come in this way to have the form of mental illness which in the originals as they are, they do not have.[38]

Clinical descriptions and methods of description are elaborated and modified as psychiatrists and others begin to frame as descriptions the types they discover in their working experience. Different kinds of practice generate different experiences and different typological knowledge. The nature of the psychiatrist's working experience is a function of how the psychiatric agency or service is articulated to the local community and its organization of access. Thus the clinical types to be found in the textbooks and journals are constructed out of the relation of psychiatry to the actualities of the community.

Psychiatry maintains a constant relation to a world which is constantly changing and constantly evolving changed situations which produce troubles coming within its jurisdiction. A change in the basis of psychiatric experience resulting from establishing a different type of agency and creating thus a new psychiatric constituency will have the same effect. Psychiatric responses to changes learned and dealt with in actual local situations appear as new clinical insights, the description of variant clinical entities, the evolvement of new methods of treatment (for example, family therapy) and so forth. The process can be diagrammed like this:

Figure 3.[39]

Psychiatric concept (e.g. depression)

↓

spelled out as clinical type in textbook (c.f. Stafford-Clark's description above)

↓

Psychiatrist in clinical setting encounters patients to be diagnosed who fit clinical type but plus something else which he can't find in the textbook or journal descriptions. ← **something going on in society that we don't know about, but it does bad things to people**

↓

Psychiatrist writes paper for journals describing depression plus x

↓

new textbook or new edition of textbook includes depression plus x as part of clinical description

These descriptions, theories and practices of therapy are not confined to the professionals. In various ways and often intentionally (an educated clientele is easier to handle than an uneducated) these kinds of information are fed into the general knowledge about psychological problems available through women's magazines, through television dramas, through courses in mental hygiene, and in Psych One Hundred, as well as into the training of professionals such as teachers, social workers, etc. In this way, my seeing my own or you seeing your experience as a matter for psychiatric care comes about from knowing how to describe it and look at it in these ways. Or my seeing or your seeing someone else's behaviour as describable in such ways. To be able to make such a description is to know how to make what I feel or you feel or she is doing, into a matter which is psychiatrically actionable. The reality of mental illness is a recycled reality.

The statistics, then, do represent something which is real about the troubles which people have, but what is real cannot be separated from the professional and administrative operations which make those troubles actionable. These operations make over, tidy up, sort out and shape what is actually happening with people into properly recognizable forms. If you are dealing with a 'well-educated' population, then much of the shaping will have already been done before the patient gets to the agency.[40] The people who are counted in the statistics are entered by these processes into a system which eliminates the situational variations, the contexts, the actualities, the recurrent social conditions characteristic of a given community, industrial structure, class system, etc. Any psychiatric agency comes to be organized in relation to a definite constituency (or set of constituencies). This constituency is in part organized by its own policies, by the uses it comes to serve and by how access to it is controlled. The book-keeping of the agencies which *Statistics Canada* compiles is the end-product of these processes. What Chesler [41] and Gove & Tudor [42] have done is to take these stripped-down bits of information and try to reattach them to the situations in which they arose; to patch them together again into some kind of simulacrum of the form they had before they went through this wringer.

V
What I think we can learn from the statistics

In returning to the statistics we are going to approach them differently knowing that what they can tell us is very limited and also that they tell it from the one-sided point of view of the psychiatric establishment. The approach we will use differs from either of those previously described (Section III) in that we will not use a causal model at all. Our last section imperceptibly junked even the modified causal model we ended up with in Section III, at least so far as the uses of the statistical information are concerned.

What we have moved towards is a way of thinking about psychiatry as a complex socially organized method of controlling types of problems which are constituted (a) as problems and (b) as psychiatric problems, in the actual processes of doing something about them. Psychiatry is articulated to problems which are shaped by the very work it does. The material it works on is what has happened and is happening to people – their experience, suffering, desperation, disorganization, as these arise in the actual lived situations. The social and economic organization of society generates typical situations for people to endure or suffer *as individuals* because they have no power to change them and do not even see them as matters that can be changed. The ordinary conditions of people's lives are given. Their determinations are beyond their control. That *is* reality therefore. They (we) work within it. There are typical locations of 'strain.' These are socially structured and distinctively formed. The corporate executive who drinks to keep himself up for his work becomes an alcoholic (perhaps) and so (perhaps) does the auto-worker who drinks desperately and convivially on Friday and Saturday nights. Such differences disappear in the diagnostic categories but their social structuring is distinct. Differences in social class provide just such actual differences in the social structuring of lived experience and the consequences of its living. (On these *Statistics Canada* is consistently mute.)

We have learned that the statistical information will not give us information directly or even indirectly about such points of strain. What we can look for, however, in the statistics are the organized practices which relate psychiatry as a process of control to those points of strain. The information which is counted up is produced as part of these organized practices and can be related back to them – though indeed only tentatively.

We will look therefore in a very straightforward and simple-minded way at what is there in the statistical data to see what it can tell us about the relation between psychiatry and the situation of women. In looking at the statistics and in describing what I think can be seen, I've tried to anchor my interpretations in an understanding of how they are produced and of the working processes which transform and create the reality they seem to record. This can be done only rather imperfectly because our knowledge of these processes and how they work is rudimentary at this time. But it's the only way to go.

When we compared the Canadian with the U.S. statistics in Section II we found some fairly marked differences between women and men in the proportions of first admissions to types of in-patient facilities. Women's share of first admissions to public mental hospitals was only 39% whereas their share of first admissions to public psychiatric units was 60% (see table 1). Public psychiatric units and psychiatric hospitals provide short-term intensive care. Some public mental hospitals do a share of this work too, but they also provide for longer term and more custodial types of care as well as greater 'security.' It is this type of difference that I want to explore a little.

The federal statistics do not include figures for out-patient treatment, but those for British Columbia do. They show a pattern similar to that reported for out-patients in the States by Chesler.[43]

TABLE 5 [44]

British Columbia: Patients resident or on caseload, residential and out-patient facilities (ages 15-69), showing percent women, 1972.

	Residential	Outpatient	Total
Women	739	3329	4068
Men	1060	2387	3447
Total	1799	5716	7515
Women as % of total	41%	58%	54%

Note: There are differences between how the B.C. and the *Statistics Canada* figures are drawn. We are looking here at caseloads or patients in residence rather than first admissions. Moreover the B.C. statistics uses an odd age range because it extends to 69, an age at which rather different factors enter in. It isn't possible to separate out those over 59 because of how the ages are grouped.

The combined figures for residential and out-patient treatment show women with a slightly larger share of the total (54%). When we look at how this total is made up, however, we find considerable differences between residential and out-patient facilities. Women are only 41% of residential whereas they form 58% of out-patient caseloads. Presumably residential facilities would correspond to those listed by *Statistics Canada* (insofar as they are represented in B.C.).

Another way of focussing the statistical information is to look at the proportions of each category in different types of facility. Recalculating the *Statistics Canada* information (from table 1) shows rather different patterns of distribution for each sex.

TABLE 6

Percentage of women and men first admissions in selected types of psychiatric facility (age 15-59), 1960.

	Percentages of all women	Percentages of all men
Public Mental Hospitals	23 (4,608)	34 (7,223)
Public Psychiatric Units	60 (11,948)	37 (7,815)
Psychiatric Hospitals	12 (2,485)	13 (2,752)
Hospitals for Addicts	4 (846)	15 (3,164)
TOTAL (100%)	19,887	20,954

Note 1: Numbers appear in brackets below the percentages.
Note 2: This time I have left out Federal Psychiatric Hospitals. This is because I'm exploring patterns of relations of psychiatric agencies to people in the community.
Note 3: This table is based on the information in Table 1.

Only 23% of women are first admissions to public mental hospitals. They are markedly concentrated in public psychiatric units (60%). If we group the two types of short-term intensive care facilities, public psychiatric units and psychiatric hospitals, we have 72% of all women first admissions to in-patient treatment.

The picture for men differs in these ways: there is little difference between public mental hospitals and public psychiatric units so far as men's first admissions are concerned (34% and 37% respectively). Combining these with the short-term intensive care facilities make(s) up to 50% of men first admissions (as compared with 72% of women). Hospitals for Addicts receive 15% of men first admissions.

The British Columbia figures can be refocussed in the same way and they too show quite marked differences between the categories of women and men.

TABLE 7

Percentage of women and men resident or on caseload in different types of facility, B.C., 1972. (ages 15-69).

	Residential	Outpatient	Total 100%
Percentage of all women	18% (739)	82% (3429)	4168
Percentage of all men	30% (1060)	70% (2387)	3447

Note 1: Numbers appear in brackets after percentages.
Note 2: This table is based on Table 5.

For both men and women a substantially larger proportion are in out-patient than in residential care. However the difference is considerably greater for women. Only 18% of women who are patients of psychiatric agencies in B.C. were in residential treatment in 1972 (which means of course that 82% were out-patients), whereas 30% of men were in residential care.

The kinds of differences that are showing up can be summarized like this: the proportions of both women and men in different types of psychiatric agency (neglecting here the differences between first admissions and being 'on the books') increases as the agencies segregate patients less from the community or can be combined with continued living in the community. But this is much more marked for women than for men. 23% of all women first admissions in 1970 were to the most custodial type of institution; 72% of all women first admissions were to the short-term intensive types; and in B.C. in 1972 82% of women in treatment were out-patients. For women the psychiatric relation appears to be more closely integrated with and does less to interrupt the continuities of their lives in the community than it does in general for men.

TABLE 8

Percentages of women and men in selected diagnostic categories, all institutions, first admissions (ages 15-59), 1970. *Statistics Canada.*

	% of women	% of men
Schizophrenic	13	14
Affective Psychosis	11	6
Neurosis	48	25
Personality Disorder	7.6	10
Alcoholism & Alcoholic Disorder	6.1	32
Percent of total in selected categories	85.7	87

Note: These are selected diagnostic categories only. The percentages are based on the total for all diagnostic categories. Complete figures and percentages can be found in Table B in the appendix.

Perhaps we can get something more out of looking again at the diagnostic differences between women and men which we saw earlier in examining the Canadian statistical information in terms of Gove & Tudor's analysis. Remember we will not be interpreting diagnostic categories as attributes of the patient prior to her psychiatric contact. How women and men are distributed in diagnostic categories is interpreted here in terms of what it can tell us about the social organization of that relation. Again we will refocus the figures as we have just done for psychiatric agencies, treating women and men as separate categories and finding out how they are distributed among the diagnostic categories. (Table 8)

As we'd expect, there are quite marked differences in the patterns of distribution for women and men. Most notably we find that nearly one-half (48%) of all women first admissions to in-patient treatment are diagnosed as suffering from neurosis as compared with only one quarter (25%) of men. Further for men the two types of alcoholic diagnoses combined make up nearly a third (32%) of all men first admissions whereas for women they form only a small part of the total (6.1%). Women are clumped in the three diagnostic categories of Schizophrenia, Affective Psychoses and Neurosis (approximating Gove & Tudor's definition of mental illness.)[45] These three subsume nearly three quarters (72%) of all first admissions among women whereas for men they make up less than half the total (45%). The corresponding grouping for men are Schizophrenia, Neurosis and Alcoholism, plus Alcoholic Psychoses (71% of the total).

Here is a tentative and summary account of what the differences in the socially organized relations of psychiatry to the situations of women and men might be:

The boundaries of being well and being sick psychiatrically are not so clearly defined for women by the social organization of psychiatry. Women's mental sicknesses are themselves not so well defined. A lot of them turn up in the vague and rather catch-all category of neurosis (48% - table 8). The proportion is likely to be considerably higher for people in out-patient treatment and in treatment with private practitioners[46] and we've seen above how women are distributed there (tables 4 and 5). Then there appears also a tendency for women's diagnosis to group into categories which focus on their emotional states. Nearly 60% of women first admissions to in-patient treatment were diagnosed as either affective psychosis or neurosis (table 8). Finally the treatment or care they receive is less of an interruption in the continuities of their daily lives in the community.

For men on the other hand the boundaries seem somewhat more clearly drawn. There are fewer in the vague category of neurosis (only 25% – table 8). There is no indication of concentration in the 'emotional' types of diagnosis. And there is this marked difference between men and women in the proportions diagnosed as suffering from some form of alcoholism. Among men this is 32% of all first admissions to in-patient facilities (table 8). Being sick seems to involve more determinate and segregative types of intervention (30% of men are in residential care in B.C. as compared with 18% of women – table 5). Perhaps for men psychiatry typically steps in after something has happened or deals with the end-products of what has been happening to men over a period of time in their typical social contexts of strain.[47] It takes some time to become an alcoholic, for example. Table 2 above shows us that the highest rates of hospitalization first admissions for men comes in the 40-49 age group whereas for women it is in the years from 30-39.

The kinds of differences that emerge are not very distinct or substantial. Perhaps we should not expect the differences between women and men to be differences of magnitude. Women and men share a common social class position and a common set of social economic circumstances. They experience and live them differently because the ways in which they come together to work and live are also the ways in which their situations and experience diverge. There are indeed different locations and biographies of strain. Psychiatric agencies are not intended to register these but to deal with them as problems within their professional and administrative scope. What we have is a sketch of a possible difference in their pattern of handling women as problems as compared with men. I think as a very general pattern, it can be articulated to the general situation of women thus:

Women are normally economically dependent. Their access to work is ordinarily to relatively or absolutely underpaid jobs. Their working conditions are generally inferior to those of men. They are under-unionized and under-represented by their unions where they are unionized. The jobs they get to do are relatively uninteresting and they do not change or progress in them over the years (what looks okay at 23 doesn't seem so great ten years later).[48] Women routinely have little money to dispose of for their own. They have little opportunity for autonomy or for alternatives to marriage or means to escape from it when it runs into difficulties. Because they have little money at their disposal they have little choice with respect to leisure activities, personal spending and the like. The hours of work in the home if they are married, particularly when the children are young are elastic and often stretched as far as they will go. Women are subject to a great deal of moral pressure through their children. Economic dependence of the mother-children unit in marriage is 'enforced' by lack of adequately paid work outside the home and alternative forms of child-care (or other forms of support). Women are socialized for submission or hardened to it – less perhaps for direct obedience in these days than for submission to an existence within these highly restricted structures of action. They do not develop themselves as physically active people. They learn not to recognize or to suppress anger. They practice passivity as an active discipline. And further, their lack of access to money means a generalized lack of access to the major means to act in this kind of society.

These restrictions are the realities of women's situation. It is a very narrowly circumscribed reality in a way which men's (at least in this society) is not. These are the "realities" as I defined reality earlier – the conditions, constraints and exigencies which can't be changed and are ordinarily taken for granted. Reality (in this sense) is drawn in a tight circle around women. The scope within which they can move is very narrow.

We've noted that for women psychiatry seems to organize their problems as predominantly emotional. Their concentration in the category of neurosis is of special interest here. Neurosis organizes (or represents an organization of) a problem for psychiatry in a determinate way. It is distinguished from psychosis because it does not involve 'a loss of contact with reality.' Reality I've suggested, for women, is this narrow scope of action and control. Being 'in contact with it' means treating it as given. The idea of neurosis focusses on the state of mind or the emotional state as the problem for psychiatric intervention. Emotional states are thus given independent status as problems. Not only are they detached from the situations in which they arise. They are also in this way disconnected from the possibilities of action. And surely that is where emotional states naturally move – into activity. In the psychiatric work, they become what has to be treated (by psychotherapy, tranquilizers, shock, and etc.). For women, psychiatry institutionalizes the divorce of feeling from doing. And it appears to do so as a routine maintenance activity, picking up and organizing as its problem a socially structured situation in which doing is radically restricted and feeling has nowhere to go.

There is one further thing to be said, however, which is not a conclusion but a necessary attention to how the agenda of this paper has been set by the statistical information. *Statistics Canada* gives you no information which enables you to say anything about differences in social class in relation to psychiatry. Nor do most other sources of statistical information. There is one major U.S. study which looks at class differences and mental illness.[49] We know from this that there are important differences between the manual workers and white collar and upper class groups with respect to patterns of care and diagnoses as well as overall rates of mental hospitalization. Some of their findings suggest bases of interpretation and analysis of the kinds of statistical information we have been studying which would break down the *generalized* patterns and show varying relations of psychiatry to women and men in terms of their social class. These patterns will have been *submerged* in the overall figures we look at. Hollingshead and Redlich show for example that their two classes of manual workers have higher rates of hospitalization for psychoses and are more likely to end up in custodial types of care, but that white collar and upper class groups show higher rates of neurosis and higher rates of out-patient and (naturally) private psychiatric care.[50] We cannot of course explore the implications of this. But it is suggestive if we think of the dominant pattern which we have been sketching for women as one that may be articulated to the situations of middle-class rather than working class women. It is important to begin to recognize what the statistics *will not* tell us.

Acknowledgement

I am indebted to Yvana Christie for typing the original draft and for many helpful editorial notations, and to Steven Smith for helping me to check out the tables.

Statistical Sources

British Columbia Department of Health, Mental Health Branch, 1972 Statistical Report, December, 1973.

Statistics Canada: Mental Health Statistics, Vol. 1, Institutional Admissions and Separations, 1970.

Appendix: definitions and source tables

Definitions, *Statistics Canada*:

Mental hospital	An institution that provides treatment for all types of psychiatric conditions and includes facilities for long-term care.
Psychiatric hospital	An institution that provides short-term intensive treatment.
Psychiatric unit	A unit within a general hospital that is organized for the treatment of patients with psychiatric disorders.
Hospital for Addicts	A facility specializing in the treatment of patients suffering from alcoholism or drug addiction.

TABLE A

All institutions, first admissions by sex & age (ages 15-59), all diagnostic categories excluding organic, senile dementias & diseases of childhood, 1970.

AGES	WOMEN	MEN	TOTAL	WOMEN AS PERCENT OF TOTAL
15-19	2,532	2,562	5,094	50%
20-29	5,418	5,444	10,862	50%
30-39	4,441	4,554	8,995	49%
40-49	3,942	4,700	8,645	46%
50-59	2,419	2,884	5,303	46%
TOTAL	18,752	20,144	38,896	48%

Description: Women's and men's shares of first admissions to all types of institutions (1970) is the same for age groups 15-19 and 20-29. Thereafter women's share is somewhat lower than men's. The greatest difference is in age groups 40-49 and 50-59 when women are 46% of the total.

Note 1: This table differs from Table 2 in the text showing rates for each age group. The *rates* include *all* types of mental disorder whereas this has been pruned in accordance with the procedures described in the introduction. For these age groups, the organic disorders, senile dementias, and diseases of childhood contribute minimally.

Note 2: This table is based on *Statistics Canada*, op. cit. Table 2, pp. 30-31.

TABLE B

All institutions, first admissions, 1970, Diagnostic class, by sex, ages 15-59.

PSYCHOSES	WOMEN		MEN	
	Numbers	Percentage	Numbers	Percentage
Alcoholic Psychoses	100	0.5	470	2
Schizophrenia	2,503	13	2,900	14
Affective Psychoses	1,966	11	1,147	6
Paranoid States	291	1.6	270	1.3
Other and Unspecified	767	4	621	3
NEUROSES, Personality disorders, and other non-psychotic disorders				
Neuroses	8,945	48	4,986	25
Personality Disorders	1,417	7.6	2,049	10
Sexual Deviation	10	.05	97	.5
Alcoholism	1,047	5.6	5,973	30
Drug Dependence	393	2.1	848	4
Psychical disorders of presumably psychogenic origin	39	.2	40	.2
Special Symptoms not elsewhere classified	59	.3	15	.07
Transient situational disturbances	1,011	5.5	731	3.6
Total (Psychoses and Neuroses)	18,548	99.45	20,147	99.67

Note 1: The percentages don't add up to 100% because of rounding.

 Note 2: Based on *Statistics Canada*, op. cit. Table 4, p. 44.

Notes:

1. P. Chesler, *Women and Madness* (Doubleday and Company, Inc., New York, 1972).

2. Chesler, ibid., pp. 119-120.

3. Based on Table 6, *Statistics Canada: Mental Health Statistics, Vol. I, Institutional Admissions and Separations, 1970*, p. 52. For the definitions of the types of institution, see the appendix.

4. Based on Table 2, *Statistics Canada*, op. cit., p. 33.

5. Chesler, op. cit., p. 120.

6. W.R. Gove & J.F. Tudor, "Adult Sex Roles and Mental Illness," *Changing Women in a Changing Society*, ed. J. Huber. (University of Chicago Press, Chicago, 1973).

7. Gove & Tudor, op. cit., p. 69.

8. Gove & Tudor, op. cit., p. 50.

9. Gove & Tudor, op. cit., p. 50.

10. *Statistics Canada*, op. cit., p. 15.

11. Based on Table 4, *Statistics Canada*, op. cit., p. 44.

12. See also, Chesler, op. cit., p. 40.

13. Chesler, ibid., p. 33.

14. Chesler is careful to restrict what she says about the data to women's "involvement with psychiatry." In other contexts she speaks of how "some women are driven mad" by being "impaled on the cross of self-sacrifice" (Chesler, op. cit., p. 31); of madness as a "rite" which women "perform" (Chesler, op. cit., p. 33); of "useless women" becoming "visible" as insane (Chesler, op. cit., p. 33); and etcetera. Generally however she takes advantage of a variant of the model I describe, and this is certainly the method of thinking which others use in interpreting what she says.

15. T.Szasz, *The Myth of Mental Illness: Foundations of a Theory of Personal Conduct* (Dell Publishing Company, New York, 1961).

16. T. Scheff, *Being Mentally Ill: A Sociological Theory* (Aldine Press, Chicago, 1962).

17. R.D. Laing, *The Divided Self: A Study of Sanity and Madness* (Quadrangle Books, Chicago, 1960).

18. Szasz, op. cit.

19. Scheff, op. cit.

20. Szasz, op. cit.

21. Scheff, op. cit., Ch. 2, pp. 31-54 in particular.

22. Scheff, ibid.

23. Laing, op. cit., Ch. 2.

24. See Chamberlin's, "Women's Oppression and Psychiatric Oppression" in this book which describes this experience. See also R.D. Laing, *The Bird of Paradise or the Politics of Experience* (Penguin Books, Harmondsworth, 1967), p. 58.

25. M. Kimball in her paper, "Sex Role Stereotypes and Mental Health" in this book describes a study by Rosenhan which illustrates this.

26. *Statistics Canada*, op. cit., pp. 14, 15.

27. It is a picture which describes the psychiatric process but it is a general bureaucratic procedure which has been fairly extensively described elsewhere. For technical descriptions and analyses see H. Garfinkel, *Studies in Ethnomethodology* (Prentice-Hall, Inc., Englewood Cliffs, N.J., 1967); D. Zimmerman, "Record-Keeping and Intake-process in a Public Welfare Agency," *On Record: Files and Dossiers in American Life*, ed. S.D. Wheeler. (Russell Sage Foundation, New York,

1969); D. Sudnow, "Normal Crimes: Sociological Features of the Penal Code," *Social Problems, 12*, Winter, 1965; A. Cicourel, *The Social Organization of Juvenile Justice* (John Wiley and Sons, New York, 1968); D.E. Smith, "The Social Construction of Documentary Reality," *Sociological Inquiry, 44*, (4), 1974.

28. Kimball, op. cit., in this book.

29. E. King, "How the Psychiatric Profession Views Women," in this book.

30. D.E. Smith, "Women and Psychiatry," in this book.

31. G. Errington, *Negotiating the Decision: What is a Police Matter?* M.A. Thesis in Sociology, University of British Columbia, 1973.

32. Sudnow, op. cit.

33. M. Spring Rice, *Working Class Wives*, quoted by S. Rowbotham, *Women's Consciousness, Man's World* (Penguin Books, Harmondsworth, 1974), p. 75.

34. R. Knight - as told to, *A Very Ordinary Life* (New Star Press, Vancouver, 1974).

35. Knight, ibid., p. 5.

36. The person is "The patient..." (It can be fitted on like a big sack over anyone's head); the clinician commands a vantage point from which he can treat both insider's and outsider's knowledge as if they were (a) equal and (b) his. The behaviour is described so that it is quite detached from the contexts in which it is lived. The terms used to describe behaviour do so as if it had no 'doer' — "there is *a* withdrawal of interest." The patient does not hesitate but "display(s) a hesitation." The terms generalize in a way which makes them capable of describing a wide range of actual and various instances.

37. Sir D. Stafford-Clark, *Psychiatry Today* (Penguin Books, Harmondsworth, 1963), pp. 95, 96.

38. Kimball's paper (op. cit.) in this book quotes examples from Rosenhan's study which illustrate the same process.

39. This is a variant version of Atkinson's formulation - J.M. Atkinson, "Societal Reactions to Suicide," *Patterns of Deviance*, ed. S.J. Cohen. (Penguin Books, Harmondsworth, 1974).

40. D.E. Smith, "K. is Mentally Ill: The Anatomy of a Factual Account," *Ethnographics*, eds. J.M. Atkinson and J. Coulter.

(Martin Robertson, Ltd., London, 1975).

41. Chesler, op. cit.

42. Gove & Tudor, op. cit.

43. Chesler, op. cit., p. 120.

44. Based on "Patients Resident or on Caseload by Age, Sex and Facility, Dec. 31, 1972," in *British Columbia, Department of Health, Mental Health Branch, Statistical Report*, 1972 (December, 1973), pp. 18, 19.

45. Gove & Tudor, op. cit.

46. Gove & Tudor, ibid., p. 61.

47. I note in this connection the observation of a woman admitted for the first time to Riverview Mental Hospital. She said:

> I was in a female ward and my observation on that was probably contrary to what you think, and that is that most of the men I met there were obviously a good deal sicker than most of the women. A lot of the women in my ward had really nothing wrong with them at all, except they got a bit overborne by home troubles, and needed a rest. Whereas most of the men I met were really freaked out.

(from an interview with Cathy Batten, a member of the Mental Patient's Association done by Eve-Lynne Rubin and accompanying her presentation at the Vancouver Women's Health Symposium, June, 1974).

48. Here is a quote from a short paper (anonymous) which describes what took place in a session with her psychiatrist of eight years when she read sections of the paper "Shrink! Shrank! Shriek!" by Barbara Findlay (in this book) to him.

> We then went on to the subject of power, and he told me that he does have power over me and that that is the thing that I dislike about him and which makes me feel angry towards him. After all I stuck to a job for eight years when I kept wanting to quit because it was dull and uninspiring, and I felt that it killed any creative energy I had in me. This has made me feel very bitter about my psychiatric experience. However, since I now know that I am not creative and brilliant and will never be a famous writer, I should be truly grateful that he has made me stick to this dull and uninspiring job.

Women's occupational conditions and opportunities are part of this general situation I'm describing and this paragraph almost caricatures the relation of psychiatry to it.

49. A.B. Hollingshead and F.C. Redlich, *Social Class and Mental Illness* (John Wiley and Sons, New York, 1958).

50. Hollingshead and Redlich, op. cit., Tables on pp. 268-270 and 210 and 212 are particularly relevant.

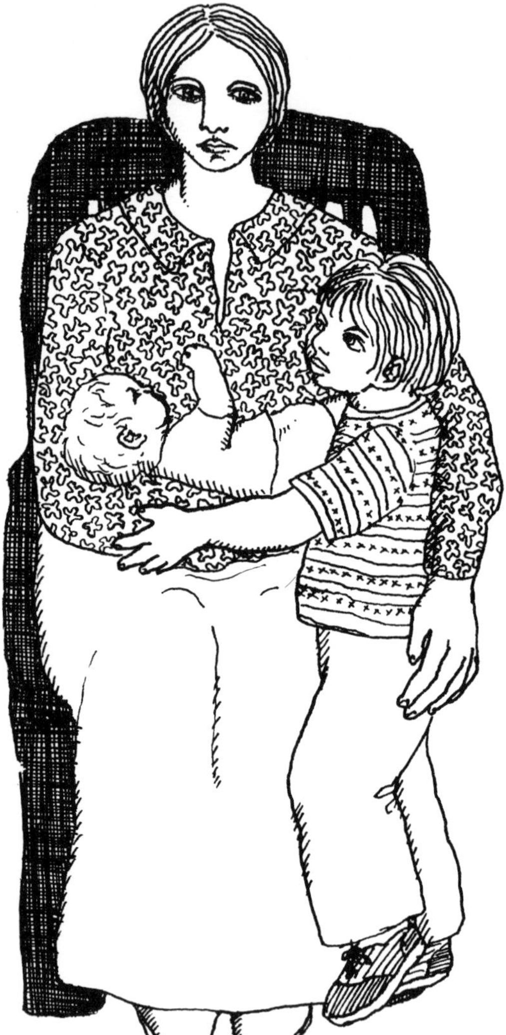

WOMEN, SEX ROLE STEREOTYPES & MENTAL HEALTH: CATCH 22

Meredith Kimball

I. Introduction

A woman is passive, submissive, dependent, narcissistic. She is a supporter of men and children. Her goal in life is to marry, have children, love others. She puts herself last: the ideal woman is self-less, thinking first of others, last of herself. She is unable to think in abstractions, she personalizes the world, she lives vicariously, through others. She is other-directed, her self-esteem is formed by what others (or important others – parents, husbands, children) think of her. Her moods are cyclical or controlled by her hormones. She is emotional, expressive, irrational, whimsical, unstable, easily distracted, unobjective, and silly.

A man is active, aggressive, independent, objective. He gets his emotional support from a woman. His goal in life is to be someone, to achieve, to leave his mark on the world. He puts his career first, he takes his family for granted. He thinks in abstractions and deals with the world impersonally. He lives for himself. He is inner-directed, has an independent sense of self-esteem. He is stable, his moods do not fluctuate, he is dominant because of his testosterone. He is unemotional, rational, determined, objective and serious.

So the stereotypes are formed. They are independent of reality. No one knows a single person, woman or man, who fits all the stereotypic descriptions of her/his sex. But the stereotypes remain with us. Children learn them early, adults recognize them easily. They stay despite evidence to the contrary. They serve, as all stereotypes do, to simplify and categorize a basically chaotic world. They are prescriptive as well as descriptive – they are the body of *shoulds* and *ought tos* as well as of *is* and *ares*. They are the myths that are created by those with authority to speak for the culture for the purpose of social control. If a woman is (should be) passive, if her goal is to marry and have children, then a woman who is active, unmarried and childless is abnormal, strange, confusing and ought to be unhappy. If a woman is passive, married, and a mother of two children, then she is normal, familiar, easy to understand and ought to be happy.

The myths, the shoulds, the prescriptive statements embedded in the sex role stereotypes of our culture affect all of us. We have learned them at an intellectual and an emotional level. We are uncomfortable with deviation from expectation. An aggressive, forceful woman is castrating. A passive, soft man is effeminate. A person may choose to accept the prescriptions for her/himself; reject them, ignore them, fight them, enjoy them; but in one way or another the stereotypes are responded to. Mental health workers are, like anyone in the culture, also affected by the stereotypes. Definitions of mental health reflect the stereotypes. This is demonstrated clearly and simply in a series of studies by Inge Broverman and her colleagues.[1] They designed a series of 122 bipolar items, each of which defined two ends of a perceived psychological continuum. Of the 122 items they chose, 38 items represented scales that were seen as descriptive of stereotypic male-female differences. Of the 38 items, 27 were male valued and 11 were female valued. A male-valued item was one in which the pole which was seen as masculine was also seen as the more socially desirable pole (ex:1) not at all aggressive – very aggressive; 2) very home oriented – very worldly; 3) almost never acts as leader – almost always acts as leader; 4) unable to separate feelings from ideas – easily separates feelings from ideas. Examples of female-valued items include: 1) very talkative – not at all talkative; 2) very neat in habits – very sloppy in habits; 3) very quiet – very loud; and 4) easily expresses tender feelings – does not express tender feelings at all.

Seventy-nine clinicians (46 men and 32 women) then participated in a study concerning perceptions of mental health. The clinicians were divided into three groups. One group was given the "male" instructions which said "think of normal, adult men and then indicate on each item the pole to which a mature, healthy, socially- competent adult man would be closer." They completed the questionnaire by checking the pole on each item which they thought more accurately described a healthy adult male. The second group of clinicians were given "female" instructions – that is they were asked to indicate the pole on each item which they thought more accurately described a "mature, healthy, socially-competent adult woman." And the third group was given the adult instructions in which they were to check the pole which more accurately described a "healthy, mature, socially- competent adult person." The results were very interesting – first of all, there were no differences between the opinions of the male and female clinicians as to what they thought was healthy for a man, a woman or an adult person (sex unspecified). There were very few differences between the description of the normal, healthy, adult male and the description of the normal, healthy, adult person. However, the picture provided by these clinicians of a normal, healthy, adult woman differed from that of a normal, healthy, adult man in being "more submissive, less independent, less adventurous, more easily influenced, less aggressive, less competitive, more excitable in minor crises, having their feelings more easily hurt, more conceited about their appearance, less objective, and disliking math and science." As the authors state, this constellation seems a most unusual way of describing any mature, healthy individual.

The catch 22 or double bind nature of women with respect to the mental health stereotypes is clear from Broverman's study. There are two standards of mental health – one for adult males and adult people, another for adult women. Should a woman change toward being a healthy adult, she becomes sick as a woman. If she is a healthy woman, she is sick as a person. The extent to which the catch 22 can extend is illustrated in an article about hysteria by Wolowitz.[2] In his discussion of hysteria it becomes clear that the clinical definition of hysteria is remarkably close to the clinical definition of normal femininity. Even the word hysteria is feminine in origin. It comes from the Greek word for uterus and for some time hysteria was thought to be caused by a wandering uterus which had come to rest at the affected body part.

The double bind exists because the standards for mental health are defined by the group in society given the authority to speak for the mental health of others – white, middle-class males. Other groups (middle-class women and women and men from different class, ethnic, and racial groups) are compared to the dominant standards. The results of this comparison for people other than white, middle-class males are two-fold: 1) a down-grading of the person in ways that she/he can be compared to the middle-class male standard; and 2) an elevation to a super human level in ways that the person has access to experiences unavailable to middle-class men. When middle-class women are considered examples of each of these two possibilities is clear. The first is demonstrated by the Broverman research. An example of the second is the pedestal phenomenon. Women have access to the experience of pregnancy and childbirth – in this and in their role as mother they have been treated as morally superior, angels, above petty involvement with the world of men. Erikson's (1964) theory of the psychology of women is based on the pedestal phenomenon.[3] This article is interesting reading because it is so clearly an example of the pedestal bias in psychological thinking about women. The most blatant example of this reasoning occurs in the beginning of his article. Erikson argues that it is *as mothers* that women should be represented in politics. Men in the striving for bigger and better weapons and wars to use them in, have created such a potential disaster that women with their natural concern for life and healing can (perhaps) change the course set by men.

> The question arises whether such a potential for annihilation as now exists in the world should continue to exist without the representation of the mothers of the species in the councils of image making and of decision.[4]
>
> Maybe if women would only gain the determination to represent as image providers and law givers what they have always stood for privately in evolution and in history (realism of householding, responsibility of upbringing, resourcefulness in peace keeping, and devotion to healing), they might well be mobilized (by whom?) to add on ethically restraining, because truly supernatural, power to politics in the widest sense.[5]

Nellie McClung in her political work with the Canadian suffrage movement long ago drew her audiences' attention to this very form of reasoning designed to elevate women to the superior position through their role as mothers and thereby keep them out of the political arena. She refers to this line of argument as "dope"

> Some of us have suspected for a long time that a good deal of the teaching of the world regarding women has come under the general heading of 'dope'. Now 'dope' is not a slang word, as you may be thinking, gentle reader. It is a good

> Anglo-Saxon word (or will be), for it fills a real need, and there is none other to take its place. 'Dope' means anything that is calculated to soothe, or hush, or put to sleep. 'Sedative' is a synonym, but it lacks the oily softness of 'dope'.
>
> One of the commonest forms of dope given to women to keep them quiet is the one referred to in a previous chapter: 'The hand that rocks the cradle rules the world.' It is a great favourite with politicians and not being original with them it does contain a small element of truth. They use it in their pre-election speeches, which they begin with the honeyed words: 'We are glad to see we have with us this evening so many members of the fair sex; we are delighted to see that so many have come to grace our gathering on this occasion; we realize that a woman's intuition is ofttimes truer than a man's reasoning, and although women have no actual voice in politics, they have something far more strong and potent – they have the wonder power of indirect influence.' Just about here comes in 'the hand that rocks.'
>
> Having thus administered the dope, in this pleasing mixture of molasses and soft soap, which is supposed to keep the 'fair sex' quiet and happy for the balance of the evening, the aspirant for public honours passes on to the serious business of the hour, and discusses the affairs of the state with the electorate. Right here, let us sound a small note of warning. Keep your eye on the man who refers to women as the 'fair sex' – he is a dealer in dope!

With the development of the women's movement, people have become more aware of the stereotypes and critical of them – as they apply to women. The stereotypes, as they apply to men, continue unnoticed. Cavanaugh (1974) used the Broverman questionnaire to study the attitudes of high school counsellors.[7] There were, as in Broverman's study, three groups of counsellors. One group was asked to complete the questionnaire for a "mature, healthy, female student"; another group completed the questionnaire for a "mature, healthy, male student" and a third group rated a "mature, healthy student." In addition each counsellor was asked to complete the questionnaire for her/himself. The awareness of counsellors to the stereotypes as they apply to women was apparent in two of the results. The first concerned the selective return rate of questionnaires. Males who were asked to rate a female student were least likely to complete and return the questionnaire.

In addition, several of those who did made hostile comments at the end of the questionnaire. One male counsellor even returned the questionnaire unanswered but with a comment that he was not going to be trapped into answering something that would make it appear he stereotyped women. It evidently did not occur to him that the questionnaire allowed a neutral or non-stereotyped response. The second result involved the ratings. Women counsellors rated a mature female student in a less stereotyped way that they rated themselves. Men counsellors rated a mature male student in a more stereotyped way than they rated themselves. It is stereotypes as they apply to women, not men, that are being questioned and are changing. This is not surprising since the male stereotypes reflect the ideals of the middle-class male.

It is important at this point to look at the definition of mental health – what is meant by mental health? The most prevalent kind of definition used is one of adjustment. If a person can adjust to, function as he/she is expected to, by society, then she/he is healthy. This is clearly reflected in Broverman's study. The therapists were judging mature, healthy men and women in terms of their adjustment to expectations we all hold for women and men, i.e. the sex role stereotypes of our society. In addition to the expectations of how people are to behave and feel, there are also expectations as to the roles people are to fulfill. Women's role is defined, traditionally in terms of being a wife and mother; men's role in terms of financial provider. In the second section of this paper, I will examine the traditional roles of women, in an attempt to show how their structure within our society makes adjustment difficult for many women.

One of the problems in using adjustment to roles and expectations as a definition of mental health is that of determining when adjustment is present or absent. The absence of adjustment is judged in one of two ways: 1) the person her/himself judges that she/he is not functioning, adjusting to what is expected and seeks therapy or hospitalization as a result; 2) someone else who has been given the authority by society to make such judgements (psychiatrists, psychologists, social workers) decides that a person is not functioning adequately and legal steps are taken to force the person to obtain treatment. In the third section of this paper, I will examine some of the information available which attempts to measure the adjustment of women and men in our society. The information draws from both self report data and from commitment data.

 An alternative definition of mental health is that of self-actualization.[8] Here the criterion is not adjustment to expectations, but the development of one's interests and potentials, the fulfillment of one's possibilities. This development may or may not take place within the traditional roles provided by the society. How and in what circumstances self-actualization can occur are determined by the individual. Self-actualization for some women may necessitate a rejection of the traditional roles of wife and mother, for others the redefinition of those roles, and for others the traditional roles provide the framework for self-actualization. What is important is to realize that self-actualization and adjustment do not necessarily go together.

Adjustment does not necessarily imply self-actualization. And self-actualization may mean lack of adjustment, pain and confusion in defining and living different roles, and the risk of social disapproval for one's actions. In the final section of this paper I will explore two forms of therapy which have, for me, focussed on the self-actualizing process. For women interested in creating new non-traditional roles in their own lives, the self-actualizing definition of mental health is a model that has advantages over the adjustment model. It allows a flexibility and range of possibilities that are not apparent in the adjustment model. It leaves marriage and children for women as a choice, it does not conflict with choices of an alternate life style, and it provides a framework for the integration of many "deviant" (as labelled by the adjustment model) roles into a healthy, full life.

II. Women's Roles and Mental Health

The roles that women are expected to fill as a part of the normal development — those of wife and mother — are so structured in our society that they present situations that are often incompatible with mental health.

A woman is expected to get married. The choice of a husband is presented as one of the most important choices she will ever make. Reinforcing this view, Erikson has said

> Young women often ask whether they can 'have an identity' before they know whom they will marry and for whom they will make a home. Granted that something in the young women's identity must keep itself open for the peculiarities of the man to be joined and of the children to be brought up. I think that much of a young woman's identity is already defined in her kind of attractiveness and in the selectivity of her search for the man (or men) by whom she wishes to be sought.[9]

Thus women are socialized to believe that their identity is dependent on whom they choose to marry and that the state of marriage is necessary for their happiness. Yet the state of marriage is less healthy for women than for men – quite the opposite to our usual views that devious women trap unwilling and unsuspecting men into marriage. Jessie Bernard in her book *The Future of Marriage* presents in detail the statistical evidence for the greater mental health of married men and single women. Thus married men as compared to non-married men have better mental health, show fewer serious symptoms of psychological distress, commit fewer crimes, earn more money, and are twice as likely to report themselves as very happy.[10] Even the two major disadvantages that men are most likely to report concerning marriage – the responsibility of financial support of the family and the sexual restrictions of monogamous marriage are changing with the increasing number of wives working outside the home and the changing moral values concerning extra-marital sex.

In comparing married with non-married women a very different picture emerges. For example, more married than unmarried women are bothered by feelings of depression, unhappy most of the time, feel they are about to go to pieces, commit more crimes, and are found to be passive, phobic, and depressed.[11] After discussing many studies Bernard concludes

> It is not necessarily the magnitude of the differences that is so convincing; it is, rather, the consistency of the differences. No one difference or even set of differences by itself would be definitive; but the cumulative effect of so many is. The poor mental health of wives is like a low grade infection that shows itself in a number of scattered symptoms, no one of which is critical enough to cause an acute episode. And so, therefore, it is easy to ignore. Or to dismiss. Or to blame on women themselves. There must be something wrong with them if they are psychologically so distressed.[12]

Bernard goes on to explain this low grade infection in terms of the experiences of the housewife: the woman upon marriage experiences a change in work, a disconnection with the outside world, she is required to make many adjustments (most couples report that the woman made most of the changes): in effect she dwindles into a wife. A woman who is perfectly capable of taking care of herself before marriage may become helpless after 10 or 20 years in the role of housewife.

It is not the state of marriage, but the role of housewife that is so destructive for women. The statistics that are available for wives working outside the home show that in most ways they are mentally healthier than wives at home. An interesting contradiction in the research occurs when we find that although married women show up worse on most measures of mental health than single women, more married women (as compared with single women) report themselves as happy. This self report goes in the face of a large body of statistics. Perhaps as Bernard argues married women report themselves as happy because they are married. Despite their real experiences in marriage, they have so long assumed that marriage will make them happy that they assume they must be happy because they are married. Perhaps the women, like the researchers who study marriage, assume that because they have made the adjustments required in marriage that they are happy. Bernard also argues that the socialization process that prepares women for marriage may "deform" them to fit marriage as it now exists – with the results that they feel they are happy because they fit the situation. They are happy because they are adjusted, normal women: i.e. they have conformed to the expectations of society. They have in their role as wife adjusted to what is expected of normal women.

The role of mother is also one that presents women in our culture with some clear contradictions. The very definition of femininity includes the state of motherhood. We read from Bettleheim:

> As much as women want to be good scientists and engineers, they want first and foremost to be womanly companions of men and to be mothers.[13]

and from Rheingold:

> Woman is nurturance...anatomy decrees the life of a woman...When women grow up without dread of their biological functions and without subversion by feminist doctrines and therefore enter upon motherhood with a sense of fulfillment and altruistic sentiment we shall attain the goal of a good life and a secure world in which to live.[14]

Women to be normally feminine must bear and raise children, yet the status that falls to women as mothers is very low and the supports provided by the social system for raising children are negligible. Mothers are told to act by instinct.

That they will know instinctively the best way to raise children. This very emphasis on instinct sets women off from the rest of society's jobs for which it is assumed that people must be trained. It also implies that women operate as mothers on a more primitive level than men or women in other occupations.[15]

Mothers are expected to be very intimate with their children, indeed be everything for them, while they are young, and then at some appropriate point to let go of their children so that the children can branch out on their own. Just as mothers are assured that their rewards for raising children will be great, they are also assured that the responsibility for everything that goes wrong with the children will also rest with them. All of this happens in the context of such a rapidly changing world that no one knows what will be the necessary qualities for coping 20 years hence.

Psychiatrists and other mental health professionals are not the only groups that put demanding and contradictory expectations on mothers. Because motherhood has been defined as the basic ingredient of femininity, issues surrounding it remain critically important for a women's feeling of self esteem. The traditional view, supported by the psychiatric profession, is that a woman who chooses not to have children is unfeminine, selfish, in short a bad person. Lois Hoffman, in discussing planned childlessness, tells how women who choose not to have children are variously described as "selfish, sick, cold and unfeminine."[16]

Hoffman argues that undoubtedly many women have had children more to avoid this negative image of themselves rather than out of any desire to have children. The women's movement in its attempt to counter the myth of motherhood, has done so largely by putting it down. Thus having children is viewed within parts of the movement as unimportant; raising children should not get in the way of the really important activities of political and economic work. No woman should consider raising children to be a full time occupation. A whole new set of myths and shoulds have been generated to support women who choose not to have children but only at the expense of women who do have children. The strength and defensiveness of the response of the women's movement is not surprising given the strength and defensiveness of the motherhood equals femininity argument of traditional society. And it is hard on an individual level to move beyond the defensiveness to a more open understanding of what the choice to have children means to young women who, at least technically through birth control, have the choice; and to a more open understanding of what the experience of having children means to women who are mothers. I have had more difficulty with women about motherhood than about any other issue that is important to us as women. I have been in several discussions which involved sensitive, intelligent, open women and seen the discussion go cold, hard and accusing when we began to discuss having or not having children. The discussion focuses on the "right" or "wrong" reasons to have children. Young women who don't want children are told "they'll be sorry" if they never have children. Older women who have raised children are challenged as to the validity of their life. When told by a woman for whom I care very much that I would never understand her because I didn't have a child and she did, I felt myself move into sadness and then into anger and defensiveness wanting to say something like, "well, you'll never understand me either." Of course the experience of having and raising a child is unique and to some extent that experience, like all unique experiences, cannot be fully understood by someone who hasn't shared the experience. Of course choosing not to have a child is also a unique experience. Most of our lives consist of unique experiences – they are what make us unique individuals. However, our feelings about those experiences are not unique but common. There is a range of human feelings which we all know – we all know fear, anger, guilt, joy, and many more feelings in some of our experiences. These we can share, and these we can understand in someone else. Doris Lessing has said it better than I can

> ... growing up is after all only the understanding that one's unique and incredible experience is what everyone shares.[17]

But we do not share the feelings in situations where they will be judged as good or bad, right or wrong. We instead become defensive, we say what we hope are right things, or the things that others have told us are right. Women need to move, especially in the area of motherhood, towards a space in which defense is not the first response, the set with which to approach the subject. Both professionals and the women's movement have not supported this move, although this appears to be changing in some places (see Lois Hoffman's article). Until women themselves can move beyond defensiveness and with self esteem and clarity claim their right to have or not have children and communicate what they feel no one (neither professionals nor the women's movement) can begin to understand what it means to be a mother.

III. Women and Mental Illness

Are more women than men mentally ill? Is adjustment for women more difficult than it is for men? If mental illness can be defined by the statistics our society keeps, it appears that more women are mentally ill. Walter Gove and Jeanette Tudor (1973) review a number of studies and report that no matter what criterion is used, more women than men are mentally ill.[18] They review community surveys, first admissions to psychiatric hospitals, psychiatric care in general hospitals, psychiatric outpatient care, and private outpatient care, and in each case there are more women using the services than men. Chesler (1972) reviews the diagnostic categories available and finds that more women then men are labelled depressive, psychoneurotic, schizophrenic, psychotic, and paranoid; while more men than women are diagnosed as having problems of drug and alcohol addiction and personality disorders (i.e., psychopathic). More women than men attempt suicide, while more men than women actually kill themselves.[19]

While more women than men are reported as mentally ill, more boys than girls are referred to child guidance clinics for most childhood emotional problems. An interesting explanation for this difference is found in the differences in the worlds of children and adults. As women and children have traditionally been grouped together, the world of childhood is a feminine one. A boy's acting out in this world appears more deviant than a girl's passivity and dependence. The world of adults is masculine. Men and women live in a world defined by men for men and women, and in this world, feminine passivity is seen and treated as deviant. Boys grow, as Chesler (1972) notes, from an opposite sexed world in childhood to a same sexed world as adults; while girls grow from a same sexed world in childhood to an opposite sexed world as adults.[20] This basic difference in the experience of the sexes is important for a person's perception of oneself as well as for the world's perception of her/him. That it is difficult to live in an opposite sexed world has been noted numerous times by educators and early childhood experts. They argue that the feminine environment of early childhood and the early school years is detrimental to boys. Much concern is expressed over attempts to change the environment. It is assumed that the environment, as much as or more so than the boy has the problem. That the adult world is masculine and that women live in an opposite sexed world has escaped everyone's attention except a few writers in the women's movement. Women have the problem, not the environment. Women are mad, poorly adjusted, mentally ill.

To judge mental illness through statistics has some major pitfalls. One is that we must assume someone labelled insane is insane. To have been in a mental hospital is to have been insane. Just how easily the labels are used in a professional setting is frightening. This labelling process has been well documented in an excellent article, "On Being Sane in Insane Places" (Rosenhan, 1973).[21] Several people, none of whom had any history of psychiatric disturbances and who had never sought or been referred for psychiatric help, voluntarily admitted themselves to several different mental hospitals. Upon being admitted to the hospital, the pseudopatients behaved in a manner which was, for them, normal. In each situation, *none* of the professional staff spotted them as normal. Instead their behaviours were seen and labelled as symptomatic of their illness. Their life histories were distorted to support the diagnosis. What is even more interesting is that in several situations some of the patients on the ward did detect the pseudopatients. They realized the pseudopatients didn't belong there, the staff never did. If a person has been labelled insane, then any behaviour can be interpreted within that definition. For example, each of the pseudopatients took notes on patient-staff interaction. In fear that such behaviour would bring suspicion on the pseudopatient, at first they took elaborate precautions to hide their notetaking. However, they soon found that the precautions were unnecessary. This behaviour, as all other behaviours, was interpreted as a symptom, and as such was seen as irrelevant. None of the pseudopatients' writing was ever looked at by any of the staff. A person's whole life can be translated to fit the assumed pathology. Rosenhan describes one man's development as follows

> ... a pseudopatient who had a close relationship with his mother but was rather remote from his father during his early childhood. During adolescence and beyond, however, his father became a close friend, while his relationship with his mother cooled. His present relationship with his wife was characteristically close and warm. Apart from occasional angry exchanges, friction was minimal. The children had rarely been spanked.[22]

In the hospital records the following case summary of this man was found:

> This white 39-year-old male...manifests a long history of considerable ambivalence in close rela-

> tionships, which begins in early childhood. A warm relationship with his mother cools during his adolescence. A distant relationship with his father is described as becoming very intense. Affective stability is absent. His attempts to control emotionality with his wife and children are punctuated by angry outbursts and, in the case of the children, spankings. And while he says that he has several good friends, one senses considerable ambivalence embedded in those relationships also...[23]

Another problem with the statistics is that they are based on definitions that are made by men. This is essentially circling back to the introduction of this article, but the point is important and I wish to make it in a different way here. Women more than men are likely to be perceived as mentally ill because the definitions of mental health are masculine. For example, it is argued that more women are reported as mentally ill because women are conditioned to be expressive of their emotions and to seek help. Men, on the other hand, are conditioned to keep their feelings to themselves and to solve their problems by themselves. So the reasoning goes, men and women experience the same distress, only women express it more. What gets ignored is that the expressiveness itself is seen (or can very easily be seen) as a sign of mental imbalance. It is outside the male defined area of appropriate behaviour and is therefore suspect. Chesler says:

> The greater social tolerance for female 'help-seeking' behaviour, or displays of emotional distress, does not mean that such conditioned behaviour is either valued or treated with kindness. On the contrary. Both husbands and clinicians experience and judge such female behaviour as annoying, inconvenient, stubborn, childish, and tyrannical. Beyond a certain point, such behaviour is 'managed' rather than rewarded: it is treated with disbelief and pity, emotional distance, physical brutality, economic and sexual deprivation, drugs, shock therapy, and long-term psychiatric confinements.[24]

Women are by definition less balanced, less sane than men. Or else they are as sane as men but not feminine. We are back to the beginning – back to the catch 22.

When women turn to the professional world for help, they find, as has been pointed out by Dorothy Smith (see "Women and Psychiatry" in this book), a world that is defined and run by men. The therapists (especially the ones with power) are men. Depending on the source, 85 to 90% of the psychiatrists are men, around 60% of the psychologists, and at the lowest rank – social workers – the situation reverses and women outnumber men. Even the women who are psychiatrists and psychologists have been trained by men, and thus many (as we saw in the Broverman study) hold the same basic views of their female patients as their male colleagues do.

Women as well as men invest the male therapist with more authority. Chesler (1971) did a study in which she looked at the preferences of patients for a male or female therapist.[25] Of the patients who expressed a preference, the majority of men and women said they wanted to see a male therapist. Married women were least likely to prefer a male therapist, while single women and divorced men were most likely to choose a male therapist. Reasons that men gave for choosing a male therapist include: greater respect for a man's mind; general discomfort with and mistrust of women; and specific embarrassment about "cursing" or discussing sexual matters, such as impotence with a woman (women seldom if ever expressed a reluctance to discuss sexual matters including frigidity with a man). Some of the reasons given by women for choosing a male therapist include: greater respect for and confidence in a man's competence and authority; feeling generally more comfortable with and relating better to men than to women; and specific fear and mistrust of women as authorities and people, (sometimes combined with statements about disliking their own mothers). Reasons given by female patients for requesting a female therapist include: feeling only a female would understand another female's problems, feeling that one could be less open and honest with men (in general fewer reasons were given for choosing a female therapist). Reasons given by male patients for requesting a female therapist include: expectations of being sexually attracted to a male therapist, which they thought would distract or upset them (almost all men who gave any reasons for requesting a female therapist were homosexual). One heterosexual man stated that he felt too competitive with men. The reasons given by men and women for their choice of a male therapist reflect the greater authority granted to men as well as the focus on male statements as worthy of respect. Reasons, when given, for choosing a female therapist, reflect their expected empathy or, in the case of homosexual men, fear of possible attraction to a male therapist. It is interesting that no heterosexual women chose a female therapist out of fear of possible attraction to a male therapist.

IV. Where to go from here: New forms of therapy for women.

This paper as well as others in this book have been basically critical – emphasizing what is destructive for women in the therapeutic process as it now exists. In this final section of my paper, I wish to offer some ideas and experiences that at best will be useful for some women and at worst will provide an encouraging note from one person's view. Many women will at one or several points in their lives need therapy. This is especially true of women who are involved in changing the form and meaning of their lives. Personal change involves, as a necessity, pain and chaos. People do change, but they change slowly. Change involves both insight and behaviour change and the two are related in a feedback cycle – insight can lead to behaviour change and behaviour change can lead to insight. Where the cycle starts is different for different people in different situations. And the cycle is repeated many times before a change becomes integrated into the structure of a person's life. For me, the insight usually begins the cycle. An example is the change I have been going through for the past eight years and am not done with yet. It concerns the expression of anger. The insight (which came when a friend stopped speaking to me for three days) was that I was completely unable to deal with my own and other people's anger. I was so unable to deal with it that I would smooth over, placate any situation so that anger would not happen. If I was angry, I repressed it (often realizing afterwards that I had indeed been angry when all sorts of fantasies of verbal aggression towards the person would occur). When someone else was angry with me, I would immediately put up all sorts of defenses and agree to do anything they asked. My stomach would literally do contortions, I was scared and I would deny, devalue, and wipe out myself in order to stop their anger. Having the insight, I began to try behaving differently. That meant several things. It meant being angry in any way that I could when I felt it. One time it meant screaming at someone and finding that he and I survived it. Many other times with other people it meant saying "I was angry yesterday when you..." or "I think I'm angry now." It also meant staying with other people being angry with me. It meant acknowledging their anger was real, was important. When someone said they were angry with me, a change for me was to take a deep breath and say let's talk about it. With the behaviour changes came new insights. For example, I began to see what my defenses consisted of, why I had them, where they had come from, and why I continued to use them. Then, in some situations letting go of them, being a little bit more open with my anger, and opening up to other people. I'm not done with the change yet and don't expect to be for some time (maybe never), but the small changes are rewarding. I am a different person than I was eight years ago and I like myself more.

External change in a person's life can be sudden; sometimes a person will choose this change, other times she may not. For example, a woman leaving (or being left by) her husband or lover may find herself living alone for the first time in her life. A woman may take a new job after many years of unemployment. The external form of her life becomes literally from one day to the next dramatically different. Yet she cannot change immediately to meet the situation. No person can. Suddenly the behaviours and the insights (ways of thinking about herself) are wrong or potentially wrong. Worse yet, she doesn't know what needs to change in her, or how to go about it. These are times (but not the only times) that a woman may feel a need for, or seek therapy. A friend of mine told me that she seeks outside help when she feels she's getting to be too hard on herself and her friends. I like that. One's life can feel so confused, impossible, and often miserable, that talking with friends no longer helps.

For women who are seeking change, or who have experienced a change in their lives, or who have become dissatisfied with their lives, it is often difficult to find a form of therapy that fits or works for them. Many women are thinking about how traditional forms of therapy should change. One idea I want to add to this thinking is how men and women in our society are socialized to approach emotional problem solving differently.[28] Men are socialized to be emotional problem solvers, while women are socialized to be emotional supporters. Men's socialization trains them to listen to a problem, offer a solution, often in terms of doing something differently, and *expect* that the problem is over. Because of the expectation, they are upset when the problem goes on, when the person comes back over and over to discuss the same problem. Women are socialized quite differently. They are trained to support, to offer encouragement, to *expect* that emotional problems never disappear overnight.They listen sympathetically, reassure the person they think he or she is OK, and are not surprised when the person returns a few hours, days, weeks, or months later in the same muddle about the same problem.

Therapy for women could do well to take more advantage of how women are socialized to deal with emotional problems.

Supportive, ongoing groups, for example, embody many of the parts of women's socialization. That consciousness raising groups came out of the women's movement is not surprising given women's socialization; and while most CR groups are not therapy groups, they are often therapeutic in process. Another important part of therapy for women is for them not to feel impatient with themselves when they don't solve their own problems easily or quickly. Traditional therapy (except perhaps for behaviour therapy) has not held that problems can be solved easily or that they will go away quickly. Traditional psychoanalysis is based on the expectation that it takes years of therapy to understand oneself. But it has assumed that problems have solutions and that to some extent how fast the solutions are arrived at depends on the degree of resistance the patient has to accepting the correct interpretation of the therapist. Traditional therapy also assumes termination – that after a number of sessions (be that 5 or 200) therapy is over.

It is possible to develop some guidelines for new forms of therapy which are designed with women's socialization in mind. I would like to describe the forms of therapy I find comfortable and outline the assumptions in these forms that I find fit. I believe that they are forms that reflect the female style of emotional problem solving. This does not mean men could not and (in the encounter form) do not benefit from the forms of therapy I choose to participate in. but they are forms that emphasize the supportive, open ended, continuous, small step, aspects of emotional problem solving. I have been involved in two very different kinds of "therapy." The first is a small women's group that I was involved in for four years. We began as a study group out of the original UBC women's group which met weekly during the 1970-71 school year. Becoming dissatisfied with the study group form we went through various forms of CR and encounter until two years ago. At that time, Jan Hermes joined the group and introduced a new style that the group operated with for two years. This technique is described in an article that appears in *The Radical Therapist* (Wykoff, 1971).[29]

Basically we met one night a week. During the meeting each woman had a specific time to work on any problem she wanted to. While one woman was "working," the others listened, offered support, commented on what they felt about the problem, and sometimes offered possible solutions. The woman who was working could accept the comments, potential solutions, etc. or not accept them. Suggestions about how to deal with specific (often day to day) problems were offered.

The woman had the choice, in a supportive, non-authoritarian atmosphere (we had no leader) to consider the suggestion. She could decide it sounded good, but the next day when faced with the situation, decide to do something different. The next week she might or might not report back on what she did. The range of problems brought to the group was wide. We all at various times, worked on issues surrounding sexuality, achievement, work, money, friendships, relationships with men, relationships with women, parents, loneliness, intimacy, etc. We were free to work on a problem when we felt the need to, there was no commitment to see a problem through to some resolution. It was assumed that problems do not have resolutions in any easy sense. Because we met once a week, the group was responsive to immediate problems – something that was important one week might not be the next week and might again be important the following week. Sometimes a woman would pass because she chose to report on a good thing that had happened. Women quit the group for several reasons – for some the group didn't meet their needs, or the form wasn't right for them, or they wanted to be on their own and felt the group was too confining. I found the form of the group useful for me. It was the place where I could work on the behaviour change part of my change cycle. I could bring a certain situation to the group and talk about alternate ways of dealing with it. I could settle on something (usually very small like how to handle a meeting I'm going to), try it, and again next week discuss how I felt about it. It was less often that my work in the group brought insight, although the feedback I got often included different ways of looking at a situation which was very useful. The group ended when several people moved away from Vancouver and continuity was lost.

To push the insight part of my change cycle I choose encounter groups. I go to encounter groups when I'm confused, feel like I don't know myself, and that too much is happening. I am more desperate and feel on the verge of not coping. Sometimes I feel this way and bring it to the small group, too. But as the feeling gets quite general – like life is too much, then I turn to encounter. What it offers for me is a chance to step back from day to day living and look at me – why do I do things as I do? How do I relate to people? What do I get out of behaving and feeling as I do? It is a chance to know myself and own what I am. Because only through owning and accepting what I am (especially those bad, disgusting parts of me) do I have the option to change. I do not participate in encounter groups very often – twice in the last four years, for the insights gained take a long time and lots of living in order to integrate them with the various parts of my life. And while the nature of insight is that it is sudden (the feeling is often one of a fog lifting, literally my vision changes, colours clear and brighten, depth is greater, there is a solidity to people and objects that was missing before) the nature of behaviour change is that it is slow, painful, full of false starts and mistakes. I work on behaviour change in an encounter group (just as in the small group I experienced insight). But the balance for me is the other way around – encounter emphasizes insight and the small group behaviour change.

In conclusion, I want to emphasize the individual nature of good therapy, what works for me won't work for everyone. Women have quit the small group and some of them have been very dissatisfied. People have left encounter groups. What women must move toward is finding, creating, and especially validating from their own authority, a therapy form that works for them. If you're seeing a psychiatrist (male or female) once a week and it works for you – it helps you to accept yourself and move where you want to go – then stay with it. Good therapy is hard to find. It is different for different women. You can't expect necessarily the first person or form you try to suit you. Don't feel guilty about quitting if it doesn't. Women must in this area as in many others, know themselves and take their own authority. Therapy is an area in which women (middle-class women in particular) have given up the authority to define their own experience. It's time to begin to take it back, try it on, live with it. And like all changes, that one's hard and slow.

Notes:

1. I.K. Broverman, S.B. Vogel, D.M. Broverman, F.E. Clarkson, and P.S. Rosenkratz, "Sex-Role Stereotypes: A Current Appraisal," *Journal of Social Issues*, *28*, 1972.

2. H.M. Wolowitz, "Hysterical Character and Feminine Identity," *Readings on the Psychology of Women.* ed. J. Bardwick. (Harper and Row, New York, 1972).

3. E.H. Erikson, "Inner and Outer Space: Reflections on Womanhood," *Daedalus*, *93*, 1964.

4. **Erikson, ibid., p. 582.**

5. Erikson, ibid., p. 583.

6. N. McClung, *In Times Like These* (University of Toronto Press, Toronto, 1972).

7. P. Cavanaugh, "Sex-Role Stereotypes: A Current Appraisal of High School Counsellors," unpublished paper, University of British Columbia, 1974.

8. A.H. Maslow, *Toward a Psychology of Being* (Van Nostrand, Princeton, New Jersey, 1968).

9. Erikson, op. cit.

10. J. Bernard, *The Future of Marriage* (Bantam, New York, 1972), pp. 18,23.

11. Bernard, ibid., p. 32.

12. Bernard, ibid., p. 40.

13. B. Bettleheim, "The Committment Required of a Woman Entering a Scientific Profession in Present Day American Society," *Woman and the Scientific Professions* (The MIT Symposium on American Women in Science and Engineering, 1965).

14. J. Rheingold, *The Fear of Being a Woman* (Grune and Stratton, New Jersey, 1964), p. 714.

15. E. Janeway, *Man's World Woman's Place: A Study in Social Mythology* (Delta, New York, 1971), p. 153.

16. L.W. Hoffman, "The Employment of Women, Education and Fertility," *Merrill-Palmer Quarterly, 20,* 1974, pp. 99-119.

17. D. Lessing, *Golden Notebook* (Panther, London, 1972), p. 14.

18. W.R. Gove & J.F. Tudor, "Adult Sex Roles and Mental Illness," *American Journal of Sociology, 78,* 1973.

19. P. Chesler, *Women and Madness* (Doubleday and Company Inc., New York, 1972).

20. Chesler, ibid.

21. D.L. Rosenhan, "On Being Sane in Insane Places," *Science, 179,* 1973.

22. Rosenhan, ibid., p. 253.

23. Rosenhan, ibid., p. 253.

24. Chesler, op. cit., p. 39.

25. P. Chesler, "Men Drive Women Crazy," *Psychology Today,* July, 1971.

26. Obviously this is true for men also; I am purposely limiting the scope of this paper to women, as the title of this section would suggest. A paper involving men and therapy, would be a very different paper and could best (and perhaps only) be written by a man. I would hope that men reading this paper would find points that are of use to them. I would also hope that they could see the places where women's experience is different.

27. People who claim instant external and internal change are interesting to listen to. One day at the beach I overheard a man talking to another man in just this way. He had been earning a large salary, owned a car, was buying a boat, etc. Then suddenly, one day, he gave all that up and changed. As he said, "Frankly, I decided to be a hippy." Now he lived on unemployment and what he and his wife could make from selling crafts. His wife was present and never said anything nor was she asked how she felt about this change. I believed his story – he undoubtedly was living on a tenth or so of what he previously made. His external life style had changed in almost every term. His concern about money had not changed at all. He spent the whole two hours I spent listening talking about how he bought a car for $100. ... how far he made an unemployment cheque go, how he lived so well without x, y, and z possessions. His concern for money had not changed, his life style centered around it. He had changed the external form not the internal worry.

28. Because men and women are socialized in our society to deal with emotional problems differently, this does not mean all women deal with emotional problems in one way and all men deal with them in a completely different way. Socialization practises vary enough that some women and some men will adopt a style not typical of their sex and that for most of us, there is a mixture of the two styles.

29. H. Wykoff, "Radical Psychiatry in Women's Groups," *The Radical Therapist* ed. J. Angel. (Ballentine, New York, 1971).

FEMALE "NEUROSIS": A VALID PROTEST

Eve-Lynne Rubin

Sigmund Freud wisely reflected that psychoanalysis "gropes its way forward by the help of experience, is always incomplete and always ready to correct and modify its theories."[1] Yet here we are in the mid-seventies, totally aware of the widespread influence of psychoanalysis on every existing field of psychiatry, and lacking a feminist analysis of Freud's theories which would more properly inform us about the nature of the society in which we live, and the effects of this society on women. Without such an analysis, we are almost incapable of understanding what has been labelled as "mental disorders" in women, or of effecting any worthwhile change.

To do proper justice to women, and to properly evaluate psychoanalysis as a therapy model for women, we must return to its originator, Sigmund Freud, and examine his work in a fresh light, especially since the neo-Freudian revisionists (of schools such as Erich Fromm, Karen Horney and Henry Stack Sullivan) who followed upon Freud's heels have only succeeded in distorting the original perceptions upon which Freud based his theories of psychoanalysis. In doing so they have frequently clouded the issues, rather than illuminating them. Though Fromm, Horney and Sullivan differ in their particular approaches to psychoanalysis, they share a common theoretical attitude. As Marcuse points out in *Eros and Civilization*, they discredit the influence of the libido, or sexual drive, in the production of neurosis; in addition, they attempt to take the focus of psychoanalysis away from the individual's preoccupation with neurosis, and relate neurosis to the larger context of society.[2] But they neglect the truly profound and deeply-rooted effect of societal conflict upon the individual's psyche. The revisionists stubbornly cling to the notion that a woman can create a healthy happy life for herself within the non-egalitarian patriarchal and exploitative capitalist political system. This is not true for increasing numbers of women, and this notion, which runs through almost all therapeutic models today, makes it almost impossible for women to receive help.

From a feminist perspective, I would claim that Freud's greatest contribution to society lies in his delineation of the effects of patriarchy on men and women, which clearly runs through his writings; not in his application of patriarchal attitudes to the treatment of neurosis, which clearly runs through psychoanalytic technique as practised by himself and his descendants. Freud showed how the libido operates within the patriarchal family to produce the Oedipus complex in both masculine and feminine form, and he defined neurosis in adults as the condition produced as a result of an inability to achieve positive sublimation of the Oedipus complex.

Freud recognized that it was necessary for both men and women in patriarchal society to acknowledge female biological inferiority in order for the Oedipus complex to develop. By discarding the influence of the libido, the neo-Freudian revisionists have inadvertently diverted the attention of psychoanalysis away from the effects of patriarchy on the production of neurosis, and more importantly, away from the relationship between the concept of female biological inferiority and the continued existence of patriarchy.

Under patriarchy, women must think of themselves as inferior; but female organ inferiority, as construed by Freud, is little more than a reflection of women's inferior status within the social organization of human beings. What Freud called "penis-envy," the new feminists rightly label "power-envy." The active aggressive power ascribed to the male role in patriarchal society is envied, justifiably, by women. In our culture, the penis is the symbolic manifestation of this active aggressive power – but women envy the power, not the penis. Furthermore, women cannot help but be in conflict with the passive receptive impotence ascribed to the female role in patriarchal culture. This takes its toll in how we perceive ourselves, emotionally, physically, and culturally. We perceive ourselves as outsiders, deprived of personal and political power, tyrannized by our bodies' birthing capacity.

When Freud defined "penis-envy" in young girls and its resultant manifestation in the castration complex, he was not challenging the role of patriarchy in the production of neurotic behaviour in women. Instead, Freud facilely suggests that when a young girl recognizes her inability to produce a penis, she acknowledges castration and "the consequent superiority of the male and her own inferiority."[3] Freud describes two rebellions which many occur in a young girl to interrupt the development of the Oedipus complex in its feminine form, thus contributing to the production of adult neurosis. First, she may turn her back on sexuality altogether because she is frightened by the comparison of her own sexual organs with those of men, *or* she may develop a masculinity complex by clinging to the unlikely hope that she will someday develop a penis. Freud maintains that the latter condition can lead to lesbian behaviour. But if patriarchy is to succeed, then Freud maintains that a third, more proper type of behaviour will occur whereby the young girl will arrive at the ultimate normal feminine attitude in which she takes her father as love-object, and thus arrives at the Oedipus complex in its feminine form.

It only remains, then, for the Oedipus complex in its feminine form to be resolved by the transference of the young girl's desire for her father to another male love-object, and the "normal healthy female" takes her place in adult patriarchal family structure able to service the needs of our capitalist society. Where this process is interfered with a neurotic female produces, then psychoanalysis steps in to ensure its continued existence.

As a feminist, I would agree with Freud that women can appear to behave in this way; but I would argue that it is extremely unfortunate for women to arrive at the third type of behaviour described by Freud, that of internalizing the values of a patriarchal family structure. The rejection of patriarchal sexuality and of patriarchally defined male and female roles which is implicit in Freud's description of the first two rebellions seems to be a valid protest, especially when the symptoms produced are recognized as powerful indictments of the powerless roles ascribed to women in patriarchal society, and especially, under advanced capitalism. Yet these valid protests are labelled as "neurotic behaviour." Psychoanalysts and most other existing therapists are guilty of the failure to recognize these valid protestations of women, or the related political indictments of our society which female "neurosis" implies.

Freud has done little more than demonstrate how socialization may occur under patriarchy to ensure that men will grow up to internalize the values of the society and that women will grow up to become oppressed by these same values, while their development as powerful autonomous human beings is thwarted. The values of patriarchy are obviously those that ensure male supremacy, values which fit so easily into Freud's concept of "penis-envy" in women and the related notion that women are biologically inferior. The degree to which neurosis as it is presently conceived occurs in men and women is largely a function of the degree to which we successfully internalize these patriarchal values. In addition, these patriarchal values function to maintain and give credence to an exploitative economy.

I, as a feminist, am aware of the value of psychoanalysis in revealing the activity of the unconscious, the effect of strife between the ego and the id, the power of the libido, and the effect of repression in the development of what we label as neurotic behaviour. But I reject the application of patriarchal values within psychoanalytic treatment. This only serves to perpetuate male supremacy and to service the needs of capitalism. Despite the influence of neo-Freudian revisionists, the end object of psychoanalysis remains to guarantee that positive sublimation of the Oedipus complex occurs in order for patriarchy to continue to function. Where patriarchy continues to function, capitalism thrives.

To help women to help themselves, then, the conflicts which we must endure under a patriarchal capitalist society must be recognized, and the symptoms that these conflicts are likely to produce must be interpreted as the symbolic expression of this society imposing contradictions on our female psyches. The symptoms of "neurotic behaviour" must be viewed in a fresh light, with the utmost respect for their valid protest against the tyranny of women's condition.

Since most men and some women involved in the clinical practises of conventional psychiatry and psychoanalysis share sexist norms and lack political awareness, they would not be the type of people which I would consider to be properly educated to help women. The sexist and pro-capitalist attitudes of the therapists and the intrapsychic approach of most therapies militate against the primary problems facing women today.

Since those conditions which are likely to produce "neurotic," and especially, "psychotic," behaviour in women stem from the contradiction of the powerless role ascribed to women under patriarchy with the desire of every human being for power and authority, then no conventional mode of therapy can possibly benefit women. Every conventional therapy takes as its major objective the re-socializing of those women (and men) who have failed to be properly socialized through their families, or through the pressures exerted upon them by society. In doing so, conventional therapies also function as a means of maintaining our present political system.

The master-slave relationship of the larger society of men and women is reinforced through the microcosm of the traditional therapeutic relationship between male patriarch and female patient. This must not occur where women help each other to grow. We have to explore together the contradictions imposed on us by our society with our prime objective being a coming into power through an understanding of the relationship between women's oppression, patriarchy, and capitalism. Presently, "therapy" denotes the relationship of the superior to the inferior, which is hardly what a coming into power for women is about.

We can no longer view ourselves as "therapists" in the conventional sense of the word, for therapists are imbued with the authority of the male power structure and service the interests of capitalism. We cannot "therapize" in any conventional manner. We are all victims of the same oppressions in varying degrees, so we can only support each other to overcome exploitation. Similarly, we can no longer view ourselves as "patients" in the conventional sense of the word, for patients have no authority. "Patients" are coerced into giving up authority to the therapists and the psychiatric institutions which serve the vested interests of patriarchal, capitalist society.

We should not be looking forward to reforms in the existing psychiatric structures, or suggesting that the solution to oppression lies solely in the development of "alternative" forms of therapy, feminist therapy among them. Alternative therapies are extremely valuable, they can help many women to move in more autonomous directions. But we should be asking ourselves the question, "Why should we have to have therapy at all?" By asking ourselves this question, hopefully we will begin to see that the solution to oppression and exploitation (phenomena which this book goes to great length to expose) lies in the struggle to bring an end to patriarchal, capitalist society. In the meantime, we continue to work with other women to develop our mutual strengths, and our revolutionary consciousness.

Notes:

1. Sigmund Freud, *A General Introduction to Psychoanalysis* (Permabook, New York, 1956).

2. Herbert Marcuse, *Eros and Civilization* (Beacon Press, Boston, 1955), pp. 248-249.

3. Sigmund Freud, "Female Sexuality," *Collected Papers*, Vol. 5 (Basic Books, New York, 1959), p. 257.

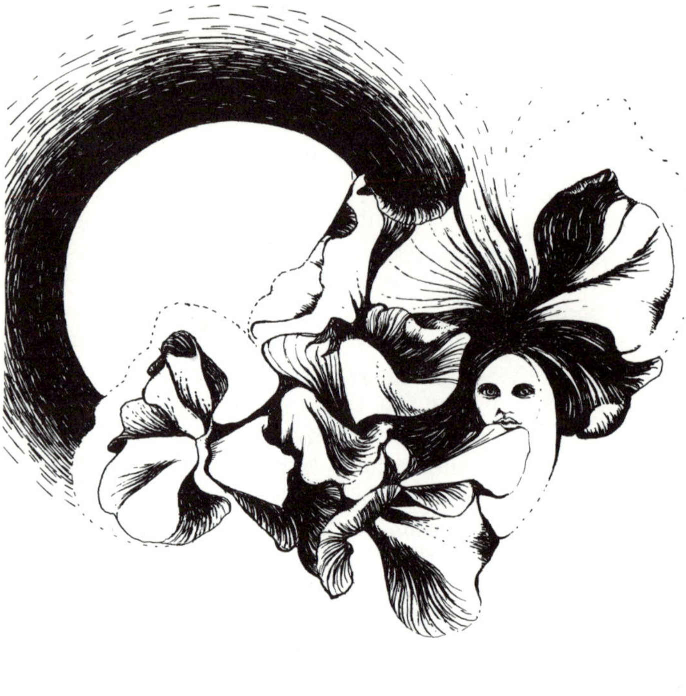

FEMINIST COUNSELLING: A PERSPECTIVE

Alison Griffith

Since the re-emergence of the feminist movement in the middle 1960's, there has been increasing awareness of dissatisfaction with all aspects of women's lives as they have been and are constituted. The dissatisfaction and questioning have resulted in a slow redefinition of our "reality" and how we see that "reality" operating within the larger social and political context.

The counselling that women and girls receive is one of the areas under question; whether it be vocational, emotional, legal, or any other of the interest areas in which counselling is involved. The underlying psychological constructs on which counselling practice is based are assumed to be gender related rather than culturally determined.[1] The attitudes and values held by counsellors and other mental health professionals were discovered to be dictated by sex-role stereotypes rather than individual capabilities and needs.[2] Testing for aptitude, interest and development was revealed as often unrelated to the actual abilities of the individual tested. Rather, the men/boys and women/girls tested were being channelled into sex-role appropriate employment, studies and behaviours. In other words, testing, theory and practice have all been found to contain sexist bias.

This, then, is the basis from which feminist counselling has begun to develop. The objective of this article is to show that it is but one aspect of feminist philosophy. To separate the two is to lose sight of the integrative basis. Also it is not sufficient to be a non-sexist counsellor. The social/political context is an integral part of feminist counselling.

Feminism is a fluid, ever-changing and evolving way of viewing and being-in-the-world. Feminism is a way of integrating the personal and the political; the masculine and the feminine. Polarities are no longer opposites in that they are no longer seen as such. Rather, they are seen as parts of the whole. They are foreground/background and may appear to be contradictory in nature. Feminist principles are co-operative rather than competitive; communal rather than individual. Feminism and feminist counselling are integrative and as such are a healing process.

Feminism assumes that the sex role identity women have been allowed has been both limiting and destructive. Feminine traits are not as valued socially as are masculine traits, [3] and as a result women have a more negative self-image than do men. Therefore, alternatives for behaviour are explored. Additional stereotypes as to how women are or should be are avoided. Through this, an understanding of women and their hopes and fears is sought.

Feminist counselling attempts to define the limits which are self- and socially-imposed and from there, alternatives are explored. Attitudes toward women as people are discussed, and, thus, attitudes toward oneself. Identification is then made, by woman as woman. Ideal versus actual self-image is re-evaluated and in the process, self-esteem.

Feminism studies and documents power relationships. Feminist counselling uses techniques which incorporate assertiveness training, peer counselling and anger workshops.

Dorothy Smith in her paper on "Women and Psychiatry" in this book discusses the concept of "authority" in the sense of women being "authors" or "authorizing" their own structures and world-view. She proposes that women are denied "authority" within the structures which society considers "valid".

> If we do not think of the term "authority" merely as identifying an external source of commands, orders, advice, etc., but in a more primary way as identifying a social structure which assigns the authorship of acts, then to possess authority is to be that person who originates and appropriates the act as hers. Women's denial (by themselves and others) of authority to themselves deprives them of the capacity to author and authorize their own words and deeds. It deprives them of the right to complain, the right to originate knowledge, to recognize and declare to one another and perhaps to men, the reality which they knew if they had only known it. [4]

So, any feminist counselling must begin by assigning authority to women. The basis from which that authority comes is our own experience, coupled with the experience of other women. Contrary to the scientific, objective mode, subjective experience is discussed and theory and practice are then fashioned to fit the experience. Commonality is the basis of feminist analysis and thus of feminist counselling.

Claiming authority for acts and knowledge proceeds from an experimental base through consciousness-raising, counsellor training at the university level and Women's Studies courses.

Women's Studies may seem at first glance to have little to do with feminist counselling. However, in keeping with the integrative nature of feminist theory it cannot be separated. It is the vehicle for dissemination of information. It is a way of reclaiming women's history; of tracing the mythology of women; of examining cross-cultural variations in sex-appropriated behaviours; of discussing the picture of women presented in the media and its implications for restricting behaviours and alternatives. By examination of these disciplines from a Women's Studies point of view, connections can be made on a political, social and personal level. The information can then be used to place the client's needs in the counselling situation within a context which includes the three levels and thus does not talk about adaptation or adjustment, but rather awareness and action.

Consciousness-raising (C.R.) is a tool which has been used by the current feminist movement for both analysis and personal redefinition. It is not therapy, nor it is counselling, nor is it political in the traditionally defined manner. And yet it is all three and more. The concept of C.R. is a way of reclaiming the authority of women. The C.R. group is leaderless, consists of 6 to 12 women and functions ideally on the three levels mentioned above. Particularly, it serves the purpose of the validation of the reality of a woman involved in the group. Personal "testimonials" are placed within the societal and political context, and it is done with women and by women. Feminist ideals of co-operation and communality are tied within the group. It becomes a safe place for women to integrate information, discard old mythologies and try out new behaviours. Because the group is leaderless, each woman takes responsibility for her own needs and for the group process. However, at the same time, she learns through the group process, what *is* her reponsibility and what *is not*. Women often take responsibility for things over which neither they, nor anyone else, have any control. This leads to feelings of guilt and inadequacy which complement the conditioned feminine sex role identity and concomitant negative self-image. For instance, women are trained within the sex role conditioning to develop skills and expertise in interpersonal relationships. However, interpersonal relationships are notoriously uncontrollable. In other words, they often fall apart. Thus the area in which women may claim or are expected to have the greatest competency is also the one with the greatest failure rate. Differentiating what we are or are not responsible for is a beginning step. Discussing relationships in terms of the three levels means that not only are guilt and feelings of inadequacy reduced, but also the responsibility is put within the larger social/political view.

In addition to Women's Studies which gives information, reclamation and analysis; consciousness-raising which integrates personal experience, analysis and validation; we must discuss the counsellors and the training they receive. Feminist counsellors are those persons who take responsibility, time and energy to bring feminist perspectives to the counselling situation. Theirs is the primary responsibility for role modelling and in this way giving authority to women's acts and feelings.

Researchers have shown that sexism exists in social work, psychology, sociology, psychiatry and of course, school curricula. It would seem to follow, then, that schools which train counsellors would also be sexist. The textbooks, training techniques and practice of counselling within the university setting would, in all likelihood, reflect the sexist bias of the society in which it is placed. Thus, the training of counsellors must include an examination of personal bias. Counsellors must be ready to look at how they give or claim authority. They must look at the practice of counselling as they are involved in it.

Mander and Rush (1974) have developed a useful framework for evaluation techniques which also proves useful in the evaluation of practice

> When I learn or invent a new technique I ask myself, is this based on concepts of segmentation or integration? Where did the philosophy behind it come from? What political stance does it take and advocate? What relationship to power does it encourage? Does it bear the stamp of class value? Does it integrate body and mind? Is it a process which will leave room for opening and balancing of our female energies? Does it emphasize the technique or the context? [5]

If the counsellor sees the situation in which she is counselling and the techniques she is using as one which integrates rather than segments; if the philosophy is egalitarian in nature; if the political stance is one which is clear about power and power relationships; if there is little or non-class value; if integration includes the mind/body dimension, (by this I mean that psychological experience is reflected on the physical functioning level and vice versa); if it is a growing and expansive process coupled with an exploration of female energies; if the content is primary, then we have the beginning of feminist counselling. It isn't an easy task to re-evaluate within the above-mentioned framework. Nor it is easy to keep a sense of clarity. It is for this reason that I have stressed the need for counselling to be within the framework of the feminist movement. That is where the ongoing evaluation occurs. That is where it is further evolved.

As feminist counselling is developing, what are some of the primary areas of focus? Feminism as integration is "healing". Thus any counselling from that perspective would by definition be a healing process. But most disciplines which have interpersonal skills and exploration of alternatives as their centre purport to be integrative and a healing process. How then does feminism and feminist counselling differ?

Marjorie Klein in a lecture at the Health Science Centre, Vancouver (1974) discussed some of the areas considered in treatment outcome and evaluation. She saw traditional counselling as tending to regard adjustment of the individual to the situation as successful healing. Feminist counselling does not. For instance, on the pain/hurting/discomfort dimension, the alleviation of these symptoms may be seen as goals in the traditional counselling situation. However, if the goal is not adjustment but rather awareness and consequent action for change, these parameters may be a healthy sign of environmental situational response. By the same token, anger in women is often seen as dysfunctional. But, for women, anger is often a sign of a healthy response to oppression, and can be used as motivation. Pain, which is definitely uncomfortable, and anger which is not a part of the feminine sex role are not automatically bad. To work in dispersing anger and alleviating pain may be merely a way of adjusting the woman to her situation rather than allowing her to grow as a person.

Women's skills in relationships with men are often stressed in the evaluation. What is not included are women's relationships with other women; the ambivalence and competition between women as well as the friendships and sexual relationships which may or may not be present. The mother/daughter relationship is paramount here.

Aggressiveness, competitiveness and anger must be explored, not condemned. As women reclaim their identity as women, not as a feminine image, anger and hostility, aggressiveness and competitiveness come to the fore. An understanding of this phenomenon and a way of using these feelings to initiate change are things with which feminist counsellors must work. To ignore or condemn is to lose the woman's interest, trust and growth potential within that counsellor/client relationship. Flexibility and personal definition are the goals.

Finally, there is the area of body-image and sensual awareness. Here there are some special problems. Ambivalent socialization results in a dual body image for most women. Female bodies are seen as both pretty and dirty. The learned sexuality is in terms of the double standard. Most counselling techniques used by feminist therapists involve some body awareness work. The purpose is to integrate the discordant messages received by women about their bodies. The assumption is that the mind/body is an integrated entity and to work on either one or the other is to again split and separate.

Feminist counselling is not hierarchical as is most traditional counselling and therapy. It is a perspective which insists that those of equal status come together to find a common ground. Thus it does not reinforce the status and power differential. Traditional therapies, although trying to be "client-centered" have not succeeded, (see, for example, Truax's examination and critique of Rogerian therapy)[6]. Values are held by both or all parties in the counselling situation. Feminist counselling, while not value-free, attempts to state openly its value system. It is therefore more woman-centered, freer of sexist bias, and more humanly oriented. No one can be free or liberated as long as anyone is oppressed. By liberating women through women's studies, consciousness-raising and feminist counselling, the human race moves slowly toward the abolition of oppression within this society.

Notes:

1. N. Weisstein, "Psychology Constructs the Female," *Woman in Sexist Society: Studies in Power and Powerlessness.* eds. V. Gornick and B. Moran. (Basic Books, New York, 1971).
2. I.K. Broverman, S.R.Vogel, D.M. Broverman, F.E. Clarkson, and P.S. Rosenkratz, "Sex-Role Stereotypes and Clinical Judgements of Mental Health," *Journal of Consulting and Clinical Psychology, 34*, (1), 1970, pp. 1-7.
3. Broverman et al., ibid.
4. D. Smith, "Women and Psychiatry," in this book.
5. A. Mander and A. Rush, *Feminism as Therapy* (Bookworks, Berkeley, 1974), p. 96. Also see, A. Rush, *Getting Clear: Body Work for Women* (American Heritage Publishing Company Inc., New York, 1969).
6. C.B. Truax, "Reinforcement and Non-reinforcement in Rogerian Psychotherapy," *Journal of Abnormal Psychology, 71*, 1966, pp. 1-9.

A FEMINIST THERAPY SESSION

Rita MacDonald & Dorothy Smith

These are selections from the transcript of a session between a woman client and a woman therapist. The client wanted to have this record of her experience made available so that other women could learn from her. Her name, the names of her husband and child have been changed so that they can't be identified. Rita MacDonald is the therapist. I (Dorothy Smith) made the selection of excerpts and wrote the linking paragraphs. They are based on many conversations with Rita.

The client's young daughter had been identified as having emotional problems. This was the reason the client came into therapy. She had recently been separated from her husband after a long period of very difficult relations with him. What we see in these excerpts from the transcript is how the client with the therapist's help identifies the social pressures which kept her in the marriage although she had ceased to love her husband and although he was violent to her both verbally and physically. Some of the pressures are moral and religious; some of them are created for her by psychiatry and the law; others are circumstantial (such as that she is an immigrant and therefore doesn't have relatives to fall back on for help). We can see in the transcript how the trap her marriage became was put together. Psychiatry has in the past helped to immobilize her in the trap. In this session the therapist helps her to substitute the authority of her own experience and understanding for the professional version and the authority of the expert.

Let me say also something about what the therapist is doing in this session. Firstly she is encouraging her client to express her anger by banging a baseball bat on a dummy. The intermittent (bang) in some parts of the text represents the thud of the bat as the client hits the dummy. Secondly, an important aspect of how the therapist works with her client involves helping her client to act out various aspects of herself and her feelings in relation to others and to herself. Sometimes the dummy represents her husband; sometimes the professionals; sometimes it is she herself against whom the client expresses her anger (at one point the therapist helps the client to objectify herself by suggesting that she put her sweater on the dummy). She can in this way enter into dialogue with herself – expressing anger against her past self for the damage she has done to herself and then acting the role in which she shows her present self the reality of the pressures which trapped her in the marriage. In this process therapist and client together codify and give social form to the client's experience.

The client has learned from her previous contacts with psychiatry to view the fact that she did not leave her husband as her psychological problem. She has learned from psychiatry to think of how she put up with her husband's violence (largely verbal) as 'masochism'. If she didn't like it, she'd leave. That's the official interpretation. Nothing that she can recall about her feelings, her values or her situation count. But she begins from their definition first for it jibes with her own sense of outrage and humiliation.

> Therapist: What's happening to you right now? You look to me to be kind of sad.
>
> Client: No, I just don't know what to think. I just feel outrage – and not just at Dick but at myself – for not seeing, because as one of the staff was saying about violence – she said if any man hit me – that would be the end of him – and how I put up with it – how I allowed myself – to endure – not just physical violence – Dick wasn't often violent in that way – but he was violent in his language – and violent in his speech – and that can be just as hurtful and just as painful as the physical violence.
>
> Therapist: So you have some pretty strong feelings about yourself – having been in that space.
>
> Client: I feel really humiliated – I really feel I let myself down.

She is angry with herself for accepting this situation. The therapist encourages her to *tell herself* why she did. In this process she begins to see how hard it was 'to take the first step' and how hard it was to hear her trap described as "You like it – you stay there because you like it".

> Therapist: How about talking to that part of your-

self that kept you there – Put your sweater on it. (LAUGHTER) – that's good – that's helpful to make that distinction! Now this is the part of you that kept you there.

Client: I just fooled myself into thinking that I was doing something for him – that I should stick with him. Many people told me a long way back that I should take off – and I didn't think it was the right thing to do. And I just let myself suffer and I don't know – perhaps Dr. .... was right in saying that I liked suffering. But I couldn't bring myself to take such a drastic step and I think a lot of women are in that situation. *They want to do something but they don't know how to take the first step – they just don't know how to go about it – and it is hard to say to them – "You like it – You stay there because you like it. You are a masochist".*

The therapist helps her to begin to look at what that meant. As she describes it, we can see the bind it locks her into. So long as she's in the situation, she's a masochist. That means she wants to be there. She doesn't want to get out. It isn't easy to imagine what it's like to be told that you *want* to be humiliated, to be made to feel worthless. In this sequence with the therapist's encouragement she begins to feel her way to defining the situation for herself.

Therapist: Linda – how does it feel to you to have somebody say that to you?

Client: Somebody did say that to me in California!

Therapist: They said you were a masochist? How does it feel to have them say that?

Client: Really dreadful. I really felt humiliated.

Therapist: O.K., can you get into that?

Client: And yet – partially she was right – because I wouldn't get out of the situation.

Therapist: But I hear you saying only partially.

Client: Well, because the other part of me felt that it was the right thing to stick by my husband – to see if I could help him.

Therapist: So there are a lot of pressures on you even when a woman is in that kind of relationship –

The therapist has to help her oppose what she has learned about herself from psychiatry and to begin to see how that was part of how her marriage became a trap.

She is angry with herself for putting up with the situation for so long. Here the dummy represents her past self.

> Client: I hate myself for allowing it to go on for so long when I knew that I could get out of it. When I had people telling me for many, many years – and you feel that you're responsible for Ann's (her daughter) little life – and you're responsible for your own (bang) nasty (bang) predicament – and your loneliness – and your lack of home (bang) and children (bang). If you'd left long ago, in Toronto (bang), when you knew things were wrong and you were always crying because he made you so miserable. (bang) Why (bang) didn't you go then? You stupid asshole! (bang!)

Now her past self replies. She tells her present self how it was and begins to describe the nature of the trap.

> Client: Linda, I did love Dick when I first met him and we were first married. But the first indication I had of things being drastically wrong was when he started to go berserk and wild and do stupid things – impulsive stupid things. And then I realized that there was something really wrong with him but I still felt it was my duty to stick by him and I had the idea that marriage was for keeps, and that I should try to help him and, if you love someone, you obviously want to help them.
>
> Therapist: O.K., so tell Linda that you had a hell of a lot of pressures on you.
>
> Client: And the other thing was that he had no money, and he had lost his job, and I felt sorry for him, and then he wanted to go to California, and I figured that maybe if he started out on a fresh base, he'd have a chance to be more relaxed and get away from his family which was bothering him.

She goes from describing her own trap to describing it for women in general. It becomes something objective.

Client: There *are* a lot of pressures on a woman, especially when you're first married, because you think, well, you've got to give yourself time to get settled and you can't make those decisions to leave a person as easily as that when you love them. First of all, there's the loving them apart from the physical love. There's the feeling of shame and a feeling of letting oneself down – a feeling of worthlessness, and I thought I should just go on trying a little harder.

Part of the trap is how she has learned to identify her value as a person with success in marriage.

Her husband's contempt and abuse had the effect of immobilizing her. And her child's problems made it even harder to break away.

Therapist: Can you tell Linda something about how the feelings of worthlessness that you got from the marriage made it hard for you to move.

Client: The feelings of worthlessness – of being told every day that I was useless, that I was not even fit to look at, that I was just no good altogether, put me in a state of feeling, well maybe that was really the case. So I became immobilized and I could just hardly get through my day's work let alone organize myself to go and see a lawyer or organize myself to move out. It was hard enough then. When Ann's problems came along, that made it even worse, because I thought I had to support her and stick to her. ... There *were* a good many reasons why I couldn't move! There was Ann for one, and the unknown quantity of what was wrong with her. And financially I had no money. Before we went to Vancouver Island I was in a strong position to move, but then I felt guilty about going because it would mean I would leave Dick with no money at all and no job.

But she still feels – or rather her present self feels – that somehow the problem is herself.

Client: (LAUGHTER) Those are all silly excuses, aren't they? (MORE LAUGHTER)

Therapist: Is that what you're feeling?

Client: Now I am! I didn't then, but I do feel now that I was just making excuses that I could at least have gotten out of it if I'd tried. (MORE LAUGHTER) Now! (TO THE THERAPIST IN A JOKING, CHALLENGING MANNER) If I'd had the strength of character I should probably have done it. I'm sure no other woman would have put up with that nonsense.

There's a marvellous sequence on the tape here which it's impossible to catch in the transcript. There's an amazing and amazed squeak of surprise in the client's "You do? Oh!" which responds to the therapist's legitimation of her own version. It's an important sequence because the therapist authorizes the client to ditch the psychiatric version and the psychiatric vocabulary which locks her into it. The therapist uses her professional authority to give it away. The client's voice becomes the authoritative voice of her experience.

Therapist: O.K. I guess what I'm trying to do is get you in touch with some of the reasons why you couldn't leave ... I think the things you said about the social pressures of trying to stay in it and all the pressures of feeling that you had to make it work and that if you didn't make it work that you would be a failure.

Client: Do you think that's legitimate or not?

Therapist: Yes, I do.

Client: (WITH SOME SURPRISE) You do? Oh!

Therapist: You don't?

Client: Well, I did at one time but you see other people have told me since then that that's just... there's a word for it – what is it?

Therapist: Masochism?

Client: No, not exactly. There's another word.

Therapist: Rationalization.

Client: Rationalization!

Therapist: Yes. So when you said there were a lot of pressures on you to keep it together....

Client: Well, there *were*! Really and truly! Yes!

Therapist: So O.K. Let's do something else. Here's all these professionals telling you that you've been rationalizing, telling you that you should have done it, you ought to have, you should have, you could have. O.K. Say something to them.

Client: Well, first of all they didn't have to live with it! (LAUGHTER)

Therapist: O.K. I really want you to tell these guys, these bastards, all the people who have been telling you what you should do.

Client: (BANGING AT DUMMY) You don't want (bang) other (bang) people (bang) to see you as a failure (bang) and (bang) you (bang) don't (bang) want (bang) to (bang) be (bang) a failure (bang) in your own eyes (bang).

Therapist: So you tell them, that group of professionals who have been telling you what you ought to have done, and what you should have done. I'd like for you to tell them that you've had quite enough feelings of worthlessness without taking on their judgments as well.

Client: I'd (bang) had enough (bang) feelings (bang) of worthlessness (bang) from my husband. Without (bang) taking (bang) on your added (bang)... I can't think of the words...judgments about my worthlessness, (bang) about my ability to let go (bang), to leave (bang) a situation (bang) that was (bang) so (bang) painful (bang) and (bang) miserable.

Her sense of the reality of her own experience has also been invalidated in her attempt to find a legal way out of her situation. Both lawyers and therapists have denied the moral and situational actualities of her life. And notice how the therapist with her next question refers to the client's own experience as authoritative.

Therapist: Does that fit Linda?

Client: Ya, it does. It's a terribly sort of difficult thing to sort out, Rita. You know, you've sort of hit the nail on the head, because it's really hard. See! You know why I have this terrific mix-up over this? It is because, when I first went to see the lawyer, Mr. ...., he said, when I asked him if I could get a divorce on the grounds of mental and physical cruelty, it would be a very difficult thing to prove and that another lawyer could just say, could use the case against me (I think I've told you this before).

Therapist: Yes. It's O.K.

Client: Against me that – in effect to ask me why did you stay with it for so long then, and put up with it for so long if it was grim: which is the case! But there are many, I'm *sure* there must be many, many women in my position who can't quite put their finger on it but who know that they did it for really legitimate reasons in their own minds, you know, at the time, but when it comes down to the hard facts afterward, they feel mad at themselves for doing it, because then they see that it was not worth the effort of trying.

The problems created for women by the matrimonial property laws in B.C. and elsewhere in Canada are real. Men know them and use them.

Therapist: But there were very few options at the time, or so it seemed.

Client: The only thing was to have packed up and gone, and you know if a woman does that she can't claim anything, and she's in a worse position if she leaves her husband than if a man leaves. Now the thing with Dick was that he wanted me to do that. He didn't have the courage to leave himself, but he wanted me to do it; and he kept goading me and goading me to try to get me to do it. And even after he had left...he wouldn't really leave. You see he kept coming back and going into Ann's room odd nights, sleeping there and I'd find him home and he'd say, "You get out, you bitch. You're the one. You get out, and you're getting no more money from me, so just get out. Take yourself and go and leave Ann and me." And I would have gone probably. But if you do that, legally you're *really* in a bad position. And I knew that and so I just didn't take any notice of him.

The therapist validates for the client her own experience and *her actual living* of *her* situation.

Therapist: O.K. So listen, I'd like you to make one, time's moving on actually – but I'd like you to kind of clear up one thing, O.K.? Which are the kinds of things which you felt legitimately kept you in that situation?

Client: I *did* at the time and in a way *I still do feel* that they did, even though I have really – what shall I say? – contradicted myself probably in the space of ten minutes, I do feel that at the time I did believe that I was doing the right thing, and I tried desparately to get the right people to help, but it didn't work! And I *was* really bashing my head against a brick wall.

The therapist sums up.

Therapist: I guess when we do things which compromise ourselves, that makes us feel very angry with ourselves. O.K.? But I think for women in particular (and this is a message I'm giving you, something that I believe) is that for women in particular there are so many pressures and sometimes so very few options. Or the options that are available are so difficult to take that it's very hard to move, and it's very hard not to compromise oneself.

Client: Right. It is.

Therapist: And so what I'm saying is O.K., I appreciate, I really hear what you're saying, when you tell me that you're angry with yourself for staying so long. You're angry for staying in a situation that was so destructive. What I'm saying is be kind to yourself in a sense and understand that, although you behaved in a way which was damaging for you, that's how it was at the time and there were very few options and there are very few options for many, many women like you.

BECOMING A NON-SEXIST THERAPIST

Sara David

In the past three years, perhaps in reaction to or as a function of the women's movement, more and more attention has been given to the negative effects of female socialization on mental health, the discrimination against women inherent in traditional psychological and psychiatric models of human development, and the negative impact of the mental health profession on women seeking treatment. I hope to elaborate on each of these and to share some ideas with you on attitudes, behaviours and intervention likely to increase effectiveness in working with female clients. I will attempt to deal both with career counselling and counselling oriented towards alleviating personal/emotional distress. While it has been my observation that adherence to traditional sex roles has deleterious effects for both sexes, I intend to focus on issues that arise in the counselling of women. I will do this both because I am convinced that women suffer more as a result of their socialization and because I feel equally certain that traditional models of therapy have been more harmful to female than to male clients.

Chesler, (1971 and 1973), points out that women are the most "treated" group in our society.[1] One can speculate on whether this is a reflection of the fact that it is more socially acceptable for women to be emotional and to explore emotional turmoil, or whether societal pressures create more conflict and stress for women, and, therefore, more emotional disturbance. In either case, increasing numbers of women are becoming angry over the painful emotional experiences they must endure and resolve regardless of whether they accept or conform to, or reject, the feminine role. In addition to being experientially unpleasant, emotional distress and preoccupation with it limits and interferes with the impact women can have on the world. If women are to move into responsible positions in political, economic, academic and other public spheres, they will require considerable assistance in overcoming the handicaps imposed by their socialization. Once they have begun to resolve inner conflicts, they will require support in withstanding the often blatant discrimination, resentment and social disapproval that greet women who attempt to leave stereotyped roles and compete in "male" domains.

Since so much of the emotional distress experienced by women is a function of social expectations and environmental factors, intervention at the institutional level is likely to have a more far-reaching impact than individual therapy. Mental health professionals, to be maximally effective, must become agents of change, or at the very least must orient women towards, and assist them in, themselves becoming more effective as agents of social change.

For example, the university counsellor can help female students by seeking to change their insitutions in ways that will make them a less hostile environment for women. The kinds of changes most likely to establish a better climate for female students would be those that change the status of women at the university: increased numbers of female faculty; equal pay and equal opportunities for promotion and tenure for female faculty members; increased financial aid for part-time students; increased opportunity for part-time study; increased day care facilities; admissions policies that do not limit enrolment by sex; active recruitment programs to encourage women to attend university and to explore traditionally masculine fields of study.

Much can be done to increase the awareness of faculty to their differential treatment of men and women. The following are a few examples of attitudes and behaviours that discourage female students.

1. Many times, faculty members ignore female students, expect little of them, or exhibit inordinate surprise at high quality work. This betrays a basic lack of respect for women and little faith in their abilities, both of which are demoralizing to the student.
2. The male student who challenges ideas and poses questions is frequently reacted to as bright and stimulating, whereas similar behaviour in female students is experienced as an irritant. The passive male student may be prodded and given extra encouragement while the passive female student is overlooked. What is implicitly communicated is that the faculty feel a greater responsibility toward and rapport with their male students.

3. At the graduate level, female students are often excluded from the colleague status accorded to their male peers. This can have enormous impact, since accepting a student as a colleague usually means making sure that the student acquires both the skills and knowledge basic to the discipline in question and the opportunity to use that knowledge once acquired. Female students are frequently deprived of one or the other or both.

Similar efforts can be made to change other community institutions and agencies to make them less sexist.

As suggested earlier, many women will need therapeutic assistance in sorting through the many problems imposed by their socialization and the many others created by their efforts to change. Community intervention is recommended not as a substitute for, but rather as a supplement to, more direct forms of treatment.

Negative Effects of Female Socialization on Mental Health

The differential treatment of boys and girls begins in infancy and continues throughout maturation and adulthood. Male children are played with vigorously, female children are treated as more delicate and fragile. Collard (1964) [2] asked parents at what age a variety of child behaviours such as playing away from home should be expected or allowed. The mothers of girls responded with later ages than mothers of boys. Goldberg and Lewis (1969) in a study of mother-infant interaction found mothers speaking to and touching six-month-old daughters more frequently than infant sons. [3] Thus norms about appropriate behaviour are communicated, both subtly and more directly, from the earliest years.

Young boys receive encouragement to explore their environment and initiate activity. Young girls are not similarly encouraged. On the contrary, their independence strivings are frequently met with apprehension and overprotectiveness. Such anxiety communicates a lack of confidence in the child's ability to handle the task at hand and is experientially quite different from attempting something new in the presence of a beaming parent expectant of success.

Since a sense of competence is developed by children through increasingly successful interactions with their environment, (White, 1960), [4] girls can only be severely handicapped by such parental attitudes. In fact, Goldberg and Lewis (1969) report that at thirteen months of age, girls are far more reluctant than boys to leave their mothers, return to them more quickly, and remain closer to them during play. When faced with a physical barrier between them and their mothers, the girls they studied cried and motioned for help, while the boys actively attempted to get around the barrier.[5] Crandall and Rabson (1960) report similar behaviour in grade school girls who were far more likely than boys to withdraw from threatening situations or seek help from adults and peers. [6] Thus girls miss out in childhood on the experience of effectiveness necessary for later attempts at mastery.

Toys, children's books, clothing, the media, the school curriculum, peer and parental pressure, and the very structure of language and thought combine to drive home the lesson that boys require experience that will expand their options, but girls must prepare for increasingly restricted and narrow roles.

At the same time that society chips away at the achievement motives of young females, it fosters their need for approval. It is the latter, more than the former, that motivates female students to perform well during grade school and high school years, when academic success is not only accepted, but expected of them. During these years, passivity, dependence and compliance which result in respect for authority, and receptivity to the ideas of others, are conducive to success.In later years things change. Success in higher education requires an ability to function, at least a good part of the time, in a more active, assertive, challenging, critical and self-reliant manner; all are behaviours that are less familiar to women and less acceptable to others. In addition, academic success is no longer sanctioned for females. As a result, conflicts between affiliative and achievement needs are heightened. Matina Horner (1972) has documented this phenomenon quite thoroughly.[7]

Before moving on, I would like to make explicit the purpose of taking the time to go back over the effects of female socialization. There are three major points that must be made, and which it is critical to keep in mind when working with women in a helping capacity.

1. As a result of their socialization, many women have developed certain characteristics and behaviours to the exclusion or detriment of others; effective treatment may therefore require helping women to expand their behaviour repertoires and behavioural options.

2. The particular characteristics women have been encouraged to develop are those that society values least; women may therefore need help in acquiring respect for those aspects of their traditional roles worthy of admiration.

3. Quite aside from whether or not these characteristics and behaviours are valued, they are less conducive than many of those foregone to effective functioning. Again, women may need help both at the level of accepting and desiring the latter for themselves and in actually acquiring them.

What remains is to demonstrate how the socialization process affects women's mental health. As suggested earlier, female socialization and societal attitudes towards women combine to undercut women's aspirations, abilities, and opportunities to achieve. Potentially competent women who hold back or withdraw from activity fail to achieve and master. Self-esteem, which is tied to achievement and the accompanying feelings of power, is thereby reduced. Reduced self-esteem in turn leads to depression, and depression to further withdrawal from activity. Years of therapy may then ensue in which client and therapist ruminate endlessly about the childhood origins of feelings of inadequacy and adult patterns for sustaining low self-esteem. The female client may then come to feel shame and guilt at her "patient" stature. In this manner a potentially productive human being can be rendered ineffective and can become riddled with self-doubt.

Problems Inherent in Traditional Models

I would like to turn now to problems inherent in traditional psychological models. Psychology as a discipline, and psychologists as mental health practitioners, have done little to alleviate the problems faced by women living in a man's world. Clinical psychology has erred by its preoccupation with individual differences and intrapsychic dynamics.

The work of eminent social psychologists such as Asch, on conformity; Rosenthal, on expectation; Milgram, on obedience and Schachter, on interpretation of physiological arousal provide indisputable evidence that social context has a greater influence than individual traits in determining behaviour.[8] Their findings, however, have had little impact on clinical practice. The "band-aid approach" of helping women to weather particular crises, and then sending them back to the environment which precipitated those crises, persists.

Psychologists have frequently studied sex differences in such a way as to perpetuate them. To some extent, the public perceive psychologists as "experts" who can assess human potential, and who understand what leads to effective and healthy functioning. As a result, many people adapt their behaviour to fit the patterns described as healthy by the "experts". This is most evident in the reliance of parents on the child-rearing "rules" promulgated by Dr. Spock, Chaim Ginott, and a variety of others judged to be authorities on the subject. It occurs more subtly among psychology students who attempt to emulate some theoretical model of the "healthy adult" and who frighten themselves when they discover "deviant" inclinations. In this manner, descriptive observations quickly become prescriptive. Since many prominent theorists – Freud, Erickson, and Bettleheim, to name a few of the worst offenders, present women in a negative light, this can be an insidious and damaging process.

The Negative Impact of Mental Health Professionals

Counsellors and other mental health professionals have been subjected to the same socialization process as other members of our society and frequently share the same stereotypes. Several studies document the double standard of mental health held for men and women. Neulinger (1968) and the Brovermans, Clarkson, Rosenkratz and Vogel (1970) studied psychiatrists', psychologists', and social workers' perceptions of optimal mental health.[9] In the Broverman study, healthy males were described in the same manner as healthy adults, but healthy females were seen as more submissive, less independent, less adventurous, less objective, less aggressive, less competitive, more excitable in minor crises, more easily influenced, more conceited about their appearance and more easily hurt. Neulinger's findings were strikingly similar. Dominance, achievement, autonomy and aggression were considered more important for healthy male than for healthy female functioning, whereas nurturance, succorance, play, deference, and abasement were rated as stronger needs for healthy females than for healthy males.

Women who entrust themselves to therapists with attitudes such as those described above are likely to get worse rather than better. The basically negative attitude of the therapist will confirm and add to feelings of inadequacy. Moreover, the therapists' definition of a healthy adult female encourages a return to the very behaviours which necessitated treatment in the first place.

In a recent study of the political effects of clinical judgment, Abramowitz and associates gave bogus clinical protocols to professional counsellors varying only sex and the political inclination of the alleged subject. The counsellors were asked to assess the psychological status of the person whose protocol they were given. Less liberal counsellors attributed greater pathology to the left-politically active female than to her male counterpart.[10]

Such biases are not confined to the personal/emotional realm. Pietrofessa and Schlossberg (1971) examined actual interviews of counsellors in training with a female client deciding between entering a traditionally "male" and a traditionally "female" occupation. They found both male and female counsellors biased against females entering masculine fields.[11]

As mental health professionals, we have an obligation to become aware of and examine any such biases of our own. The process of change is a difficult one requiring encouragement and support. We cannot offer these without changing our concepts of what constitutes health, and of what roles and careers are appropriate for men and women.

I'd like to go back to an issue that I touched upon briefly earlier. I feel this is a point that requires much more consideration than it usually receives, because it is one of the biggest blocks in treating women. I am referring to the fact that theories of personality and therapy generally use concepts that are more or less pejorative depending on whether the focus is optimal personality development or psychopathology. Theories which rely on the latter feed into and escalate women's negative self-concepts by encouraging them to think of their behaviour in terms of abnormality and illness. This can be more upsetting than the behaviours and feelings themselves. Women can add to their self-critical arsenal labels such as "neurotic," "hysterical," and "masochistic." They can be accused of "labelling" instead of problem-solving, which, improperly handled, results in further self-denigration for being a poor client.

Many therapists who do use psychoanalytic terminology may have very positive and accepting attitudes about their clients. These therapists generally feel absolved since they can attribute increased client distress to "projection". Again, such labelling does little to solve the problem. There is a responsibility not to feed into self-doubt. The therapist must develop a language which undercuts negative labelling. The task becomes one of enabling individuals to examine their particular patterns for diminishing self-esteem without implying, and without allowing them to infer, that they are being criticized or blamed.

Because women who seek treatment are even less self-accepting than women generally, because they have had past experiences with patronizing counsellors and therapists, and because many models of therapy use negative language, this issue is likely to come up repeatedly. If the therapist is able to assist women to become more curious about but less critical of their behaviour, a quicker shift to problem-solving can occur.

Improved Therapy

Successful therapy with women requires a fundamental belief in their abilities to function well in all situations, and to take on and fulfill responsibilities in all the same areas as men with equal competence. Even women who may be currently floundering can learn to function more effectively and it is our job to help them do so.

Female students generally seek personal/emotional more than career counselling. The reverse is true of male students. Since frequent success in a field of interest can do more to elevate self-esteem than any amount of reassurance, support, or rumination, counsellors should stress the importance of career planning.

In so doing, it is important to suggest consideration of factors such as income, status, power, opportunity for advancement and change. Too frequently women are so grateful to find work and especially work they enjoy, that they overlook all of the foregoing.

Therapists need to inform female clients that many of the problems women experience are societal in origin and that society continues to exert pressures likely to maintain such conflicts. This is necessary both to undercut self-blame and to increase women's awareness of the need to seek social as well as personal change.

To this end, therapists can increase effectiveness by increased efforts on their own part to intervene at the community rather than the individual level.

Above all, the therapist must remind the client of, and continually focus upon, her resources and strengths. This is important because women have so long focussed on inadequacies that they forget about their strengths. To the extent that they lose sight of genuine skills and abilities, they will not use them.

By way of example, let me tell you about a client in one of my groups who used to frighten herself by focussing on the possible negative outcomes of any situation. The client in question had been separated from her husband for a year and was contemplating the alternatives available for interpersonal interaction. She felt terrified at the prospect of being entirely alone, imagining that she would be depressed and unable to function if she didn't have reassurance and support. She also feared establishing another primary relationship because she felt she would be a burden to her partner because of her excessive dependency. In addition, she also feared she would rely on her partner to take care of matters she could handle herself and thus become more ineffective and less autonomous. The idea of multiple relationships was also frightening because there would be too many complications.

We spent thirty minutes brainstorming all of the potentially exciting outcomes of each of these three alternatives. Soon her confidence in her ability not only to manage or cope with these situations, but to make any one of them a positive experience replaced her former fear. She bought a sailboat, learned to play tennis, became involved in schoolwork, read poetry and learned to live happily alone. She subsequently became involved in a primary relationship with a man – allowing him to meet many needs, share some activities, but at the same time maintaining her own activities and interests.

Because women experience so many of the same conflicts, I feel that working with them in groups is more effective than individual counselling. Such groups must be more than a place to ventilate and more than a place for support. Ventilation and support are both necessary, perhaps even on a long term basis for those trying to change in a world that would have them stay the same. Ultimately, however, women need more than just that. They need a place to acquire and practice new skills such as assertiveness, self-reliance, expression of anger, confrontation, and achievement. Women in groups can not only encourage and affirm such behaviours but can serve as role models for each other. The group can also provide an arena where women can learn to be more discriminating in their use of valuable emotional resources such as compassion, nurturance, warmth, and gentleness which are otherwise so vulnerable to exploitation.

Finally, without in any way withdrawing emotional support, we must encourage our female clients to channel more and more of the energies they have reserved for relationships and introspection into activity and mastery in public spheres.

Notes:

1. P. Chesler, "Patient and Patriarch: Women in the Psychotherapeutic Relationship," *Woman in Sexist Society: Studies in Power and Powerlessness*. eds. V. Gornick and B. Moran. (Basic Books, 1971), and *Women and Madness* (Avon, New York, 1973).

2. E.D. Collard, "Achievement Motive in the Four-Year-Old Child and Its Relationship to Achievement Expectancies of the Mother," (Ph.D. dissertation, University of Michigan, 1964).

3. S. Goldberg and M. Lewis, "Play Behaviour in the Year-Old Infant: Early Sex Differences," *Child Development, 40*, 1969.

4. R.L. White, "Fundamental Early Environmental Influences on the Development of Competence," *The Third Western Symposium of Learning: Cognitive Learning* (Western Washington State College, 1974).

5. S. Goldberg, op. cit.

6. V.J. Crandall and A. Rabson, "Children's Repetition Choices in an Intellectual Achievement Situation Following Success and Failure," *Journal of Genetic Psychology, 97*, 1960.

7. M. Horner, "Femininity and Successful Achievement: A Basic Inconsistency," *Roles Women Play: Readings Toward Women's Liberation*. ed. M. Garskof. (Wadsworth Publishing Company, Inc., California, 1971).

8. S.E. Asch, "Studies of Independence and Conformity: A Minority of One Against a Unanimous Majority," *Psychological Monographs, 70*, (9), 1956.

S. Milgram, "Some Conditions of Obedience and Disobedience to Authority," *Human Relations, 18*, 1965.

S. Schachter and J.E. Singer, "Cognitive, Social and Physiological Determinants of Emotional State," *Psychological Review, 69* 1962.

9. J. Neulinger, "Perceptions of the Optimally Integrated Person, A Redefinition of Mental Health," *Proceedings of the 76th American Psychological Association*, 1968.

I.K. Broverman, S.B. Vogel, D.M. Broverman, F.E. Clarkson, and P.S. Rosenkrantz, "Sex Role Stereotypes and Clinical Judgments of Mental Health," *Journal of Consulting and Clinical Psychology, 34*, (1), 1970.

10. C.V. Abramowitz, S.I. Abramowitz, H.B. Roback and C. Jackson, "Differential Effectiveness of Directive and Nondirective Group Therapies as a Function of Client Internal-External Control," *Journal of Consulting and Clinical Psychology, 42*, (6), December, 1974.

11. J.J. Pietrofessa and N.K. Schlossberg, "Counsellor Bias and the Female Occupational Role," *Woman in a Man-Made World*. eds. N. Glazer-Malbin and H. Waehrer. (Rand McNally and Company, Chicago, 1972).

EMOTIONAL SELF-DEFENSE GROUPS FOR WOMEN

Sara David

Changes in the status of women and the roles they are seeking to play in modern society have necessitated rapid attitude and behaviour change on the part of a large number of women. Mental health professionals are being asked increasingly to facilitate such change.

In 1973-74, while at the Counselling Service at Simon Fraser University, and in 1974-75 through the Departments of Continuing Studies and Interdisciplinary Studies, I initiated a series of Emotional Self-Defense Groups for women in which the elements of personal growth groups, consciousness-raising groups, communication skills groups and assertiveness training groups were combined.

The groups were open to female students, staff members, and off-campus women. There were nine groups in all, with 10-20 members in each. Most of the participants were functioning adequately and showed no evidence of gross or chronic psychopathology. However, all of the women reported some feelings of distress, or felt in some way impeded in their personal and professional development as a function of being female.

The decision to call these groups "emotional self-defense" groups was deliberate. Women face a hostile world that discriminates against them and that mounts massive pressure to force them into roles that have been societally rather than self-defined.

From infancy, women are conditioned by the toys they are given, the books they read, the clothes they wear, the media, peer and parental expectations, the schools they attend, and finally themselves, to be supportive and subservient both in marriage and in the economy. They are carefully prepared to be the facilitators who make it possible for *others* – usually husbands and children – to be the initiators of action and the decision-makers of society.

As a result of their socialization, most women have overdeveloped certain attributes such as warmth, compassion, tenderness, intuitiveness, nurturance and flexibility at the expense of certain others equally important for effective human functioning, for example, assertiveness, endurance, initiative, industry, risk-taking and self-reliance.

Women's emotional "talents" are constantly exploited and abused. The concept of "emotional self-defense" implies increasing one's awareness of, and resistance to, emotional manipulation and blackmail. This does not mean giving up the very valuable aspects of the traditional female role. On the contrary, when women are the recipients of the warmth, understanding, and support they have given to others, they come to value these functions more fully. In addition, when they begin to contrast the appreciation they are accorded when they give support to other women with the lack of response frequently experienced from the men with whom they have been involved, there is an almost overwhelming recognition of their interpersonal oppression. The result is a more selective use of their psychological resources.

Participants in these groups discover that much of the inner turmoil they may have believed was theirs alone is shared by large numbers of women. Common themes emerge. I would like to turn to some of these patterns so that those of you who work with women are alerted to watch for them and become better able to help your clients see and understand them.

As suggested earlier, many of the problems women experience are by-products of being other-directed instead of self-directed. It seems appropriate therefore to begin with an examination of the problems inherent in the development of the former to the exclusion of the latter. Since the support services women perform are taken for granted and not fully acknowledged by the recipients of those services, women are frequently unaware of the extent to which they subordinate their own needs to those of others. Since society sanctions such self-sacrifice, many of the women who are aware of it come to experience it as virtuous rather than oppressive. These attitudes are shaped at such an early age and are so deeply rooted that it takes even those who wish to do so considerable will and dogged determination to change them.

Definition of Self by Others

a) One of the most serious problems faced by the other-directed woman is that she can frequently be manipulated by language. This particular difficulty is usually discussed at great length with many personal examples introduced and explored by group members. Most behaviour can be described neutrally, negatively, or positively. By giving up the power to define what is occuring, women allow themselves to be pushed and pulled at the mercy of significant others. For example, false humility and self-effacing behaviours are encouraged by labelling them "modesty"; "submissiveness" and "acquiescence" are maintained by renaming them "flexibility" and "co-operation". Other behaviours important for individual growth but inconvenient for family and friends can be discouraged in a similar manner. For example, self-confidence, assertiveness, autonomy and independence can be viewed as arrogance, aggressiveness, selfishness and indifference. Often such negative labels are used with no malicious intent. They may simply result from the significant others not being used to such behaviours in the woman who is undergoing change. However, the effects can be equally devastating regardless of the innocence or perniciousness of the intent. Women need to be on guard against these tendencies in others (and in themselves) to sabotage the acquisition of needed behavioural options.

b) A second very serious problem mentioned when discussing the effects of abandoning the power to define oneself is that it can lead to profound self-doubt. A woman in a dependent relationship with a person who is highly critical of her may come to believe the negatively assigned characterization. Her own perceptions and intuitions can be sufficiently undermined to lead her to doubt her judgment and even sanity. This can lead to a very serious emotional upheaval.The usual way of handling such distress is to seek individual counselling or psychotherapy. The choice of the person to work with at this point can be critical. The female patient, more vulnerable and other-directed than ever, gives power to still another authority figure who is entrusted to validate or invalidate her judgment.

1. *Careful management.* When the patient has ample ego resources, this can result in rapid restoration of equilibrium. However, if the counsellor is wittingly or unwittingly sexist (or otherwise incompetent), the disequilibrium period may be needlessly prolonged.

2. *Need for approval.* Another problematic side-effect of being other-directed is a strong need for approval. Many women come to feel they must be liked by everyone, and,

similarly, are obliged to like all others. Failure to meet this impossible standard leads to feeling hurt or guilty. It becomes difficult to express resentment without profuse apologies, explanations, justifications, and sometimes tears. Similarly, criticism becomes difficult to hear, let alone evaluate, without feeling hurt, tearful, defensive or angry. Once a high level of intimacy and trust has been established, the group provides an excellent setting for becoming experientially aware of such dilemmas and for developing and practising more effective ways of handling them.

A strong need for approval can be hazardous in another way; it may lead to losing touch with skills and abilities. The high school student who stopped volunteering answers to math and science questions in order to get more dates may forget she ever had a talent in the area. The female athlete who withdraws from volleyball to be a cheerleader may never develop her own athletic skill and competence. Moreover, the strategy of abandoning basic desires to accommodate another can only have a negative outcome. Either one wins the sought-after approval for being someone other than oneself, or there is a double loss of having sacrificed self-development without having gained the desired appreciation and validation.

3. *Relationships.* Lois Hoffman (1972)[1] and Matina Horner (1972) have clearly delineated the difficulties women have balancing affiliation and achievement motives.[2] The affiliative domain is one of the few society assigns to women, and one of the few where women are not penalized for achievement. However, achievement in the realm of relationships can be thwarted by an unco-operative or intransigeant other. Nonetheless, the large majority of women persist in holding themselves entirely responsible for the success or failure of relationships. The awareness that it takes two to relate is simply not taken into consideration by many women in deteriorating relationships. Although the Simon Fraser groups were composed of bright and talented women whose presence in a university community would suggest an orientation toward academic achievement and career development, an inordinate amount of time and energy was spent in discussing relationships, problems emanating from them, the pain experienced in terminating them, and the fear of being alone.

4. *When the other fails.* One of the major tasks of the other-directed individual is to encourage others to succeed. If self-esteem is dependent on the success of a mate or children, en-

couragement may turn into pressuring and nagging a recalcitrant other. Moreover, there is a risk of defining oneself as a failure should the other fail to succeed. Because there is more direct control over one's own endurance, motivation and ability, it is far better to invest one's energy in one's own success than requiring it of another.

5. *Artificial dependencies.* Another similar problem inherent in the excessively other-directed role is that if self-esteem is based on the successful support and nurturance of others, it becomes necessary to be needed. Thus artificial dependencies may be promoted. Mothers may do many things for their children long after the latter are able to do them on their own. Since independence training is considered important with male children, the result may be a particular infantalizing of daughters. In the Simon Fraser group this issue frequently came up in broader discussions of how to balance self-development (personal and professional) with mothering.

These last two problems taken together exemplify quite clearly the double-bind conflict society has built into the female role. If children and spouses succeed they will be less dependent on the mother/spouse; if they do not succeed, she has failed. There are endless similar double binds inherent in the female role. If she is herself a success, this threatens her spouse; if she does not develop interests and abilities of her own, she becomes a bore.

6. *Physical appearance.* Because women's status and success is judged by whom they marry rather than by what they achieve, their physical appearance takes on great importance to them. In turn, to the extent that women are preoccupied with their appearance – whether it is with feeling shame about some aspect of it or with expending energy to improve it – they are distracted from learning the skills necessary for effective independent functioning. For this reason, it is best if discussions of appearance are kept to a minimum. It is a more efficient use of group time to divide it between the unlearning of ineffectual, self-defeating, frustrating behaviours and the practising of ones that are likely to be more potent.

Once women have overcome some of the major blocks discussed earlier, they can turn their attentions to action and to preparing strategies for handling some of the behavioural responses that typically greet those attempting to move out of stereotyped roles – responses such as patronizing laughter, being ignored, being misinterpreted or more direct retaliatory put-downs. In general, I have attempted, and feel it would be most useful for others doing such groups, to focus on presenting new and challenging ideas in an assertive, persistent manner which is neither attacking and accusatory nor apologetic and defensive.

There was a considerable range in the nature of the experiences participants had while in the groups and in the changes in self-concept and behaviour that occurred. For some women, the groups produced food for thought; for others, there was increased self-esteem and appreciation of other women; others became more politically active or more involved in their academic work.

One incident occurred in the fall semester that represented a fundamental shift in thought and behaviour for the individuals involved. A graduate student in psychology approached the group to fill out a questionnaire designed to assess their perceptions of men and women. She wished to determine whether their views of men and women would differ from those held by the various segments of the population sampled by Broverman et al[3] in their appraisal of sex-role stereotypes. The participants, initially willing to co-operate, found themselves unable to complete the questionnaires. They made comments such as "There are too many items for which each end of the scale is equally true," "Individuals differ from one another so greatly that I can't really make statments about all males or all females," "I couldn't fill this out even for myself because my own behaviour is different at different times and in different contexts. Choosing a point on a scale would mask this." It was the group leader's impression that three months before, these same women would either have been unaware of anything wrong with the questionnaire, or would have found the task difficult without being able to articulate why, and that in either case they would have completed it anyway.

There are a number of other indications that the group had an impact on the individuals who were in them. Two of the group members organized a women's caucus on campus. Two others formed a group called "the ad hoc student committee for women's studies on campus" which itself became a women's studies course and conducted a survey of the student body to assess student interest in a women's studies program at the University; one member was elected as the student representative to Senate; another became active in the formulation of a union for support staff – the Association of University and College Employees; and another became an ombudsperson in the existing staff association.

If in spite of their socialization and all the obstacles in their paths, women are going to continue to expand their roles, support services such as the above-described emotional self-defense groups must be offered more extensively.

Notes:

1. L. Hoffman, "Childhood Experiences and Achievement," *Journal of Social Issues, 28*, (2), 1972.

2. M. Horner, "Femininity and Successful Achievement: A Basic Inconsistency, " *Roles Women Play: Readings Toward Women's Liberation*, ed. M. Garskof. (Wadsworth Publishing Company, Inc., California, 1971).

3. I.K. Broverman, S.B. Vogel, D.M. Broverman, F.E. Clarkson and P.S. Rosenkrantz, "Sex-Role Stereotypes: A Current Appraisal," *Journal of Social Issues, 28*, 1972.

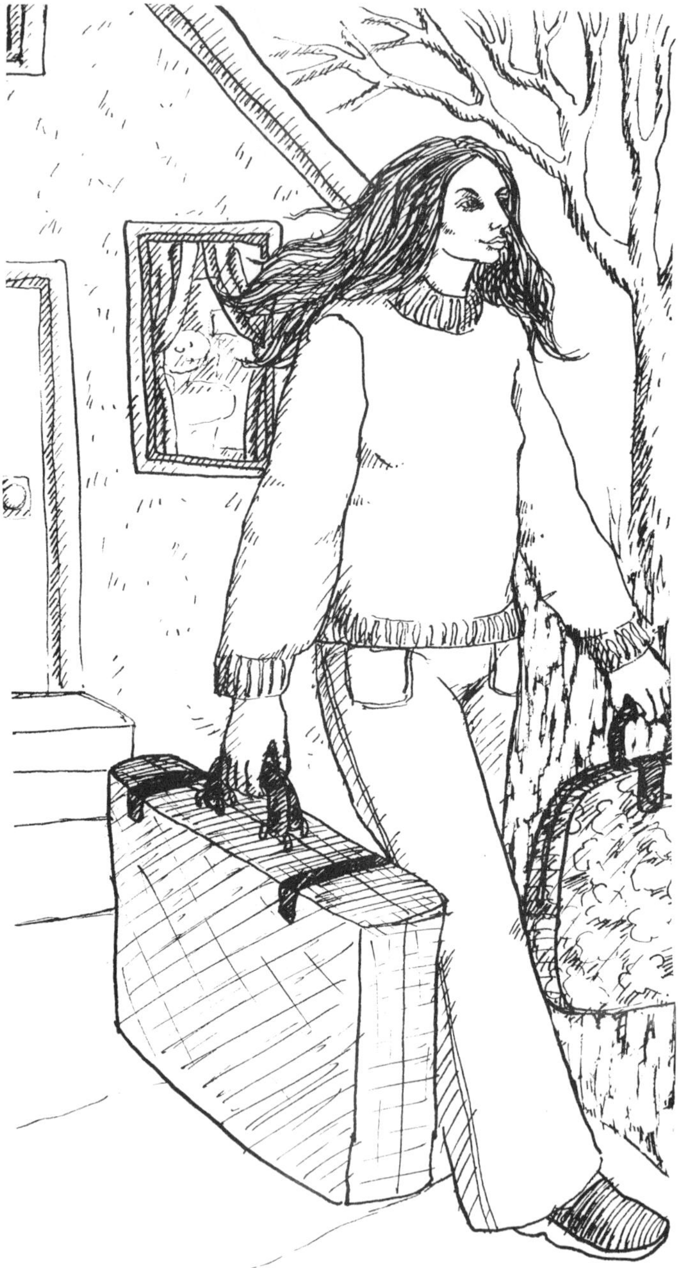

I'M NOT CRAZY AFTER ALL

Barbara Joyce

My feminist therapy began in 1970. At that time, I knew nothing of the Women's Movement, only that women's liberation really scared me; I had believed the accounts in newspapers and on television showing "women's libbers" as hysterical bitches who burned bras and made ridiculous scenes at fashion shows. Since I had had to deal with enough criticism from men, I felt I did not need any more. Life was tough enough without women's liberation. At the time I entered therapy, I was a 26 year old first-year student at Simon Fraser University. I was enjoying not being married any more and marvelling at the relative freedom of academic life as compared with that of the home and office. But I had come down fast and hard in the Financial Aid Office while struggling with the limited finances available for working-class women seeking post-secondary education. My two-year struggle to keep my marriage together had just ended in failure. My nine-year office "career" had ended with my being classified as an "unemployable" file clerk/ typist. Canada Manpower and Welfare categorized me as "crazy" because of my "personality problems." In addition, I was just starting to pull out of the worst stages of a "nervous breakdown" which began, rather ironically, only weeks after the wedding. And it was now apparent that because of financial difficulties I would also be a failure in my attempt to educate myself. I had married at 24, ("almost an old maid," as my father had constantly reminded me) and had expected to be rewarded for "finally doing the right thing." However, it had soon become obvious to me that there were more thorns than roses surrounding my marital cottage, and I had sought help in the only way available to working-class women: my general practitioner had referred me to one and then the other of the two psychiatrists who were then designated to serve the Port Coquitlam populace. So my knowledge of therapy had been limited to the stone faces of these two hard cold psychiatrists, who had told me to quit competing with my husband (I,too, had wanted to go to school), and to wash out the toilet when I was depressed. When I rejected this, I then resorted to paying a Catholic marriage counsellor who told me to stay home and be a good wife. This I tried to do until I ran out of money. At this point, I knew nothing of the human potential movement, of group therapy, or of feminist therapy. I had made constant visits to the Financial Aid Office, and when I discovered that they had no money for me, I cried. My tears were abhorrent to them so they made a quick phone call and ushered me down to the Student Counselling Service for "help." From my past experience with psychiatry and therapy, I had no reason to believe that I could get any help there, but I had nowhere else to turn and I couldn't stop crying. So here in Student Counselling I met Anne Cubitt. She was to become my therapist. She was the first person I had encountered in the past two and a half years who really wanted to know why I was crying. We set up a series of appointments, and I began my feminist therapy.

My new therapy, my real therapy, my feminist therapy was a road where "madness" did not exist, where my pain was acknowledged and where responsibility became a social and political issue, not just my individual problem. Its orientation centred on MY unhappiness and on MY powerlessness in THIS political structure, and contrasted strongly to the orientation of traditional psychiatry towards the preservance of the status quo – which meant solely my adaptation to marriage and to family life) or my PUNISHMENT for failing. My feminist therapy was gentle and patient. It encouraged my openness and growth, not my self-negation. Its process was one of strengthening me, not of defining me. It supported my change, not my adjustment. I was validated without judgments. I was nurtured without guilt. My awareness increased as my reality was confirmed. The boundaries of my feminist therapy were not determined by a scale of months, by office walls, nor by a cash exchange. My therapy involved studying Freudian misconceptions and neo-Freudian abuses. We went past Freud, through the double standard for normalcy and happiness, past family relationships towards an understanding of society. I studied sex-role stereotyping, and I was supported as I moved towards an understanding of our patriarchal society, which lays restrictions on the role of the woman and the function of the family in our culture. With this, I learned to understand the design of the role of the husband and father and of the psychiatrist, which is to restrain and punish women who wish for or struggle for self-determination. I studied feminist theory and was supported in putting this theory into practice. I learned that my oppression is women's oppression. I learned how to believe in myself and in other women. I learned about our powerlessness. Most importantly, I learned about power.

When I first met Anne, I reacted to her in the way I had learned to react when first presented with the idea of women being capable: I doubted her. When she walked out of her office to greet me, she was dressed casually. She had soft blonde hair, happy, clear blue eyes and a huge smile, and she appeared to be a lot younger than I. She was physically quite a contrast to what I had been taught to perceive as an authority, in other words, as valid. Even her office environment was different to those of my past therapy experiences. Her desk was not the usual intimidating wall for the therapist to hide behind; it was pushed up against the wall, out of the way, irrelevant. Often, one or both of us would sit on the floor and we'd kick off our shoes. Other times, we would stroll around the campus and sit on the grass. Her person became real as she talked about herself, told me of her likes and dislikes. I perceived Anne to be genuine not because of her "authority" but because of her realness.

In the beginning, I saw her twice a week; later on, once a week. During the second year of our therapy, we saw each other every two weeks. I could indicate if I needed to see her more often, and Anne would meet my demand. For a large part of this time, I was also in one of Anne's therapy groups. If confusions or problems arose in the group, we would discuss them in private sessions and would talk about different ways of helping me to make my needs clearer. In this way, I learned to use group therapy as a "safe" practice ground to help relate to the outside world.

In our private sessions, we at first talked about my most immediate problem, which was how confused I felt about my own perceptions, which had been brought into crisis by my marriage. I told Anne briefly about my family and marital history. I was surprised to hear someone say that they believed me. Anne believed me when I said that my difficult financial situation threatened my studies. She believed I had experienced feelings of unhappiness and despair during and after my marriage. She believed that these feelings were well-founded, and she said that they were shared by many other women. She brought me articles by women who felt the same way. To my great relief, we established that I was not alone, that these feelings were not "unreal" or "wrong" but that they were commonly experienced by many women. I started to consider the possibility that I was not mad.

But it took several months of therapy before I could really start trusting Anne. My past experience had taught me to be very cautious. I was very afraid that I would start needing her, and that one day she would come in and give me the standard one-sided psychiatric parting: "Okay, you don't have to come in anymore." However, after many boxes of tissues and many months of crying, I finally accepted Anne's statements that I had good reason to be sad; that I was quite right in my perceptions of my unhappy childhood and marriage. This was such a relief after the usual condescension I had encountered when I had questioned the "myth of the happy childhood" and the "myth of marital bliss." Anne helped me to realize that I was not whining, as the psychiatrists had stated; that my feelings of being unloved were legitimate. We had established that I did have some power, the power of communication. And we had established the validity of my feelings and needs. It was then that I felt I could start to trust.

When Anne asked me questions about myself, it was always in an easy, understanding manner; she would lean toward me and look me kindly in the eye. It was a question, not a demand. She would ask and really wanted to know "how I felt;" about myself, about my marriage, my husband and my family, my work and education. Did I feel powerless in society? Yes, I felt powerless! And I needed to say these things, these things that I felt, without being criticized or told that my perceptions were wrong, or that I didn't really feel those things at all, in other words, that I'm mad. First I needed to be understood. Because of her patience and kindness and interest, I felt she cared to understand.

Anne showed me that her experience of me was quite different to my image of myself which I had learned in our male society. She did not experience me as a bitch, (bad or mad wife), as did my husband, as did the psychiatrists and as did the other me. It was here that I picked up the first threads of understanding how my conflicts led me to have a "nervous breakdown." I learned that I had personality characteristics usually described as good (strong, normal) in men and described as "unpleasant" (neurotic, abnormal) in women. I learned that I had mistakenly expected men to take me seriously. Looking at my relationships with male peers in childhood, it became evident how I had clung to this expectation for so long. In my "tomboy" childhood and puberty, I stood equal to my male friends. I somehow perceived this type of relationship as "real" and I inadvertently expected the same respect in marriage (the myth), even though my other adult experiences in offices and schools indicated otherwise. I learned to be disappointed and then angry at men whom I saw as peers, for not taking me seriously. And for this reaction I was labelled, as are other women, a bitch and a man-hater.

Anne and I practiced various techniques to develop constructive ways for me to be introspective and analytical. I learned to trust in my perceptions. For example, I would tell her how I perceived an interaction in the t-group and she would either confirm it or say why she perceived it differently. I was surprised when I soon learned that this phase of the women's movement was four years into its upsurge, that the women's movement is by no means a new struggle, that the bra-burning imagery had little to do with our liberation, and that the main issue was our lack of power over our lives. I learned why my perceptions and experiences had no validity in the male social order and that this was the reality behind my serious depression. But Anne knew, she believed me and she understood how I felt. I was not crazy after all! What a relief!

We paralleled the conflicts I had felt as a child with those I had experienced as a wife. Because my earliest memories were of humiliation and punishment, the process of going over my childhood was very slow and painful. Just as I had been humiliated and denied by my parents in childhood, so had I been humiliated and denied in my marriage by my husband and by psychiatrists. I had been made powerless first by my family, and later by my husband. We saw that the character traits ascribed to the good child, traits which had been created by my father's demands, were almost identical to the character traits of the good wife, traits which had been formulated by my husband's demands. These traits were passivity, receptiveness, servility, attractiveness, pleasantness, and hap-hap-happiness. I had lived in situations where I had little or no control, and my protests were at first labelled childish and later neurotic. I became confused and learned how to turn my anger in and hurt myself. But with Anne, I learned that I was not imagining my feelings of inferiority and worthlessness at all. Servile behaviour had been demanded of me from very early on in my life. One of my previous psychiatrists once asked me to list my good characteristics. I was bewildered, and being unused to talking about myself, and very unused to a man being interested, I wanted to please him, and came up with one – I had a good complexion. He grunted in disgust. When Anne first asked me to list my good characteristics, I told her the same one. However, unlike the psychiatrist, she did not respond in disgust, but rather she looked hurt. She slowly, gently, started helping me to reconfirm myself and regain pride in myself and my womanliness. She showed me that many of her character traits were similar to mine. These are characteristics which are particularly highly developed in women, made necessary for survival in our oppression, traits which are necessary in our role as nurturer. I began to feel pride in my – our – sensitivity, perceptiveness, patience, gentleness, caring – in other words, openness. She supported me to regain a pride in my intelligence and my wit. These qualities had caused disastrous scenes during my marriage and I had sought to destroy them in my confused reaction during my depression. For fear of reprisal, I had stopped speaking almost completely. In confronting the conflicts, I learned not to punish and humiliate myself for these qualities, that in total these were qualities of strength, qualities of wholeness. They were not bad although men feared them.

What had been achieved at this point was that I was now able to see myself as a whole, not as an unconnected scattering of parts with mind and body, thoughts and emotions, separate. There was certainly still a lot of work and building to be done, but at least I now had the semblance of a foundation. And because we discovered that I was real and not crazy, we started putting my early family experiences into a social and political perspective that would enable me to liberate myself from self-blame and guilt. We did this in several ways; through my studies at university, through my work environment and through my relationships.

The first method was through my course of study at the university. I was learning to apply my new awareness and curiosity to real life. In my courses in English and Psychology, I studied women's roles. I was eager to broaden my knowledge, and Anne's role as "therapist" enlarged as my needs did. She helped me to select reading material on sexism and offered to go over my essays and discuss them. She even gave me the name of a good librarian who could help me learn to use the library.

 Soon after that, I began to see the importance of the role

of mother and the function of motherhood. We talked about this role and I began to understand that the family, especially the mother, is society's scapegoat. She is helplessly unable to totally fulfill all the emotional needs of the various family members, but is expected to do this. As a child within this type of family structure, I had looked solely to my parents for fulfillment, and especially to my mother for honest love and nurturance. Given her other chores, and given that society offers most mothers no help, she was unable to do this.

As a child, I did not understand that my mother had been given an impossible task, that the family structure is set up so that the children cannot look elsewhere for fulfillment. So I felt that it had something to do with a lack in me, and I learned how to feel guilty for that lack, and I learned how to feel worthless. As my nurturer, my mother, did not properly nurture me, I therefore perceived myself as not worth nurturing.

In therapy, as an adult, I started to understand my mother's plight. She had been trying to run a home and feed a family in poverty, with my father often unemployed. She was trying to create order whilst also caring for my father's senile parents, who were unaware of time, place or bladders. It brought about my understanding of her fears, almost dying in all her five childbirths, all of them unwanted or at least years premature. I now know her desperation for peace in a domestic structure designed to police her. It is understanding how a love she felt for one man had so completely changed her life as to be always determined first by her husband, and secondly by her children – with her own needs seldom met. It is understanding now how she could scream and tear her hair for want of a day without family pressure or worries. It is now believing that there was a lot of time even when she had no time for my fears or my needs. I understood that she did her best and when she could barely keep her sanity, she at least gave me respect of my person and my privacy.

From that understanding, I then learned that the phrase "good mother" is a contradiction in terms. A good mother raises her children in complete happiness; in other words, she has good children. One rule is, "A good mother never leaves her child alone." What this ensures is not the goodness of mothering but a constancy of policing the child and the constancy of policing the mother through her role as supervisor. So I learned why my mother went crazy; she went crazy trying to be a good wife and mother. I learned that society was driving her crazy with its impossible demands, and there were no alternatives for her. It soon became apparent just why I too had been driven mad. I was supposed to be preparing through my role as the good wife, to be a good mother. There seemed to be no alternatives for me either.

Though my family experience proved otherwise, I had clung to the myth of the happy marriage as I had clung to the myth of the happy childhood. I had rationalized these contradictions with another myth, that of individualism. In my mind, I knew that MY marriage would be different, just as I had previously wanted to believe MY childhood had been happy. So I married and my husband expected me to be a good wife, even though we had discussed having an "equal" marriage. Being a good wife meant doing the washing, ironing, shopping, cooking, cleaning, budgeting, entertaining, while continuing to smile and smile. My husband told me when to be home, which was all the time except when I was at the office, and he told me that I could have as friends people who were his friends. I didn't like it. I didn't think it was equal or fair, or that I should pretend to like it. I felt trapped. I felt like a failure. Anne and I realized that because I had shown my unhappiness to my husband in a demonstrative fashion, he had punished me by labelling me a bitch and a nag. With the help of psychiatrists, I soon began to feel like one. I drank more and more and became more and more depressed. Anne helped me to realize that my dissatisfaction with marriage was valid and that my resultant depression was my only desperate alternative at the time. We saw, by analyzing behaviourisms permitted women, that the mistake I had made was showing my unhappiness (bitch), stating my unhappiness (nag), and protesting my unhappiness (mad).

In therapy, it became clearer why I had been forced into marriage. I had been forced into marriage to gain my parents' approval and society's approval. I had only secretarial skills and a working-class background which gave me limited economic independence. The average woman works only a few years (usually in service jobs which are the lowest on the pay scales) before she is expected to marry, and stay home and raise children. In other words, she is expected to reproduce. Her relationship to production is indirect Her job is to completely care for the worker (husband) and to raise future workers and mothers. She is the slave labourer. She is on no payroll and has no workers' rights or privileges. She has few tools with which to fight for her freedom. The patter of little feet and the stomp of two big feet coming home every night is her reward.

I did not want this reward.

With these realizations, I was now able to bring things together more clearly. Like most other women, I had been in conflict with the role which I inherited from my mother. I broke out of this role when I ended my marriage, but I did not have the support or strength of conviction to see that I had been right. I had had to suffer through a nervous breakdown in order to gain strength and the desire to fight for control of my own life.

Anne helped me to form new relationships. In sessions, we talked about new people I was meeting and working with. There were many fine people whom I admired and respected. I had been avoiding these people as I felt shy and vulnerable, afraid that I might be rejected by them. I was also afraid that I was attracted to them for negative reasons. Anne and I would sit down and go over everything I knew about each person, the things they did, the things they said, and how they related to me. And if we decided they would be good for me, then Anne would encourage me to get to know them, and I did. In fact, I started forming some of my deepest and richest friendships at this time.

As my relationship to a man had been central to causing crisis in my life, Anne and I worked carefully and thoroughly as we discussed my sexual relationships with men. I felt quite incapable of recognizing sexism. I soon learned that sometimes I would let myself get into a relationship with a man although that was not really what I wanted. We carefully analyzed conversations and behaviourisms. Anne and I would go over ways in which I would "let the man win" in discussions and conversations. One time, when I described my confusion at the same point in an ongoing discussion I was having with a man, we wrote down in a little book that I carried with me three alternative statements which would stop the game and return the conversation to some type of communication. I used these phrases many times. For example, in discussions on women's oppression, the topic would often be challenged with, "But men are oppressed too!" I learned to respond with,"Yes, but that's not the point." I had spent enough time worrying about men's oppression.

With Anne's support I started taking control of my body. I was learning to question my most basic oppression; the assumption that because I had a womb my worth was to conceive and birth and unquestioningly rear and nurture. For me, it became unnecessary to keep future birthing possibilities open "just in case I might meet a man who would want me to have his child"; I did not want to be loved for a function of my body. It appeared that neither my financial situation nor our social structures would change soon enough for me to take part in rearing my child free of the hindrances I had experienced. My health was being ruined by current methods of birth control, and it was my experience that the interest of the medical industry was not, in fact, my health but rather my illness and birthing process. As I now realized I did not want to become a mother, and as I wanted to limit my future contact with the medical profession, and as current birth control methods are dangerous, I felt the safest method was sterilization. I was referred to a gynaecologist who worked with the Vancouver Women's Health Collective, spent many months discussing this "final" and "permanent" act, then had a tubal ligation. Anne was beside me when I came out of the anaesthetic. I have never regretted the decision, in fact I feel like a weight has been lifted from my shoulders.

My therapy carried on long after I decided to leave the university. Anne knew that I wanted to find some type of work that was meaningful to me. A friend of hers told her about a new mental patients' liberation and anti-psychiatry group named the Mental Patients Association* which was new and had job openings. Given my past experience, I identified strongly with this cause. I wanted to work there, but my work history was disastrous. Anne knew that I was scared, so she helped me write a resume and together we practiced the things I should say when applying for the job. I was scared at first, but delighted when I was elected. I was also very fearful that I would get fired, as had happened to me many times previously. We talked of my keeping a journal of my work endeavours, as I felt that I needed to be able to prove that I was working. So I did this until I learned to accept that at MPA I had some credence, that I was doing my best, and that everything was O.K.

While working at MPA, I made friends with women who had suffered the indignities and cruelties of mental institutions, who had had their freedom withdrawn and their minds fried with electroshock treatments or psychotropic drugs. When I heard their life stories, it became apparent that in various ways they had also been expressing unhappiness about their life situations. Instead of being helped to learn the tools for change, they were punished for demonstrating their unhappiness by being labelled "mad" by psychiatrists, being taken from their homes, which made them unhappy, and being put in mental institutions (prison) which could only create greater unhappiness.

It was then that I learned why some people see psychiatrists, some people are jailed in mental institutions, while others seek help in the human potential movement and in feminist therapy. It has to do with money and education, in other words, with class background. If I had not gone to university, I feel sure that I would never have had the opportunity for feminist therapy. Before then, I was in the same situation as millions of working-class women who are stuck in small towns all across North America. I knew only of psychiatrists and mental institutions. The connections with both were controlled by my family doctor. Like other working-class women, I lacked the knowledge that alternatives existed and of how to seek alternate help. But if I had known even then, I still probably would not have been able to pursue the strengthening and enriching processes available in the human potential movement. It is still very much, because of finances and location, a middle-class movement. Feminist therapy, women re-affirming women, crosses class barriers, and I am confident that in a very few years the same type of help that was available to me will be available in even the smallest of towns and to the poorest of women.

Looking back now, it seems obvious that I could not fulfill the needs and expectations of my husband. I know now that besides my obvious unwillingness to completely subordinate myself for a successful marriage and for approval of society that differences in our class backgrounds made it even more difficult. I had made the mistake of marrying out of my class and I didn't even understand about class divisions then.

I had grown up in a small wasp town completely cut off from the big city and any culture. My mother was raised in skid houses as her labourer father wandered through the towns of the Alberta oil fields looking for work. My own labourer father, until his marriage at 31, spent most of his life with his retired parents in a Fraser Valley homestead almost completely cut off from society. I was raised with the expectation that being a typist rather than a waitress was the most that I should expect from life. In contrast, my husband was brought up to expect to get his doctorate and work for the German diplomatic corps. His father had been a high-ranking government official and had selected his wife from a convent, judging her on her beauty and her knowledge of social skills. They were of the declining rich. So, unknowingly,

I had become socially mobile through the only means available to women – marriage.

I came to understand these differences through seeing my mother-in-law in her home. Her role was, through her home, to reflect to society the material and cultural successes of her husband. She and her home were to be beautiful and gracious and refined. But I remember seeing the set of her jaw and defeat in her eyes as she did her housework.

As my parents had not had aspirations towards high social standing, I had not been trained "how to behave" with people from "good" families. I unknowingly failed at this, and my husband hated me for my working-class background. I understand now that he felt trapped. I, who was to be the domestic symbol of his success, had become the symbol of his failure. I was hindering his social status. I had read Osborne's *Look Back in Anger* and saw that even though class backgrounds had been reversed in my case, the example of class antagonisms was still clear. For both husbands, who paid lip service to freedom, had found it easier to ridicule the wife as a powerless representative of a class rather than to organize and fight for change.

Anne's and my therapeutic relationship ended when we acknowledged our friendship. For a while we lived together, sharing the same house. This we did until our domestic needs became different. Probably what's most important is that both of us haved moved on and grown, have realized that the truest form of therapy is friendship – where each other's growth and change is encouraged and respected, and where we support each other to apply our own powers towards enrichment and the growth of sisterhood.

* The Vancouver Mental Patients Association was formed in 1971, and is a self-help group consisting primarily of ex-mental patients. It functions as a participatory democracy offering an alternative mental health service. MPA seeks social reform, and an end to psychiatric abuses and the illegal incarceration of people into mental insitutions.

Contributors' notes:

JUDI CHAMBERLIN is a former mental patient and a full-time activist in the mental patients' liberation movement. She has been a member of Mental Patients' Liberation Project (New York City), Mental Patients' Resistance (New York City), Mental Patients' Association (Vancouver, B.C.), and Counter-Psychiatry (Bellingham, Wash.). She is currently writing a book about the mental patients' liberation movement.

SARA DAVID was born in 1943 in Winnipeg, Manitoba. She did her B.A. in French and English at the University of Manitoba; her M.A. in Education at the University of California at Berkeley; and her Ph.D.in Clinical Psychology at Duke University. She has been active in the women's movement, women's studies and feminist therapy in Vancouver. Sara is currently working at Simon Fraser University.

MARSHA ENOMOTO – I've been a social worker for the past 6 or 7 years and have been active in the Women's Movement. A frustration of my work is that I see many, many women afflicted and sick with their own condition of powerlessness. A woman mental patient becomes a small part of a tight hierarchy system designed to run smoothly. The hospital may on rare occasions brutalize a woman, more commonly it protects her from the outside world, but rarely does it help her find and use her power. I cope with such frustrating aspects of my life by studying karate, but I've no similarly simple solutions for women with mental problems.

BARBARA FINDLAY – When I wrote that article my paranoia about having it published under my own name was still fairly strong, and I vacillated a lot about whether I should remain anonymous. But I have moved since then and I feel that I want to put my name to it. It would be a contradiction of the article itself to publish anonymously. Women must not be ashamed or afraid of what male society can do to us. The experience was in the first place an attempt by male society to make me accept my prescribed place. If I were to publish that account anoymously I would be giving in to the power structure that was responsible for my whole experience with psychiatry in the first place.

ALISON GRIFFITH – born September, 1942. Lived in B.C. all my life. Degrees – B.A., maj. Psychology – Simon Fraser

University. Worked in the women's movement for 4 years. Counsellor and group leader counselling for post partum depression. Coordinator, counsellor and programme developer for a woman's centre. Staff person for B.C. Women's Studies Research Centre.

BARBARA JOYCE was born in 1943 in New Westminster as there was no hospital in Port Hammond. She waitressed from age 14 to 17 while attending high school. For the next 9 years she picked up minimum wage pay cheques in various Vancouver offices for smiling, wearing a 12-hour girdle, pounding a typewriter, tottering in high heels, and putting various sheets of paper into various folders. She attended Simon Fraser University in 1970 and 1971 at the end of its political purge. She was fired from a bookkeeping job in 1971 for paying women equal wages, and since that time she has worked in the anti-psychiatry and mental patients' liberation movement, studied for a year at the Vancouver School of Art, and now works in women's publishing.

MEREDITH KIMBALL did her Ph.D. in Psychology at the University of Michigan. She has been involved in developing and teaching in the Women's Studies program at U.B.C. since 1972. Her main interests (and publications) are in the areas of the development of sex roles and achievement motivation in women.

ELINORE KING was not available at the time of publication

RITA MACDONALD – I received a Masters of Social Work from U.B.C. in 1970. For the following four years I was employed by the Department of Mental Health specializing in family and child therapy. From December, 1973 to May, 1975 I served as a Commissioner on the British Columbia Royal Commission on Family and Children's Law. I am currently serving as a consultant to the Provincial Co-ordinator, Status of Women.

EVE-LYNNE RUBIN – I was born in Winnipeg, Manitoba; moved to London, England in 1966 after finishing a B.A. degree at the University of Manitoba. In London I worked variously as waitress, book-keeper, clerk-typist, usherette, poodle-washer, shoe clerk, school teacher, motivational researcher, editor; and as a secretarial assistant to a company of science journalists, I was given increasingly more assignments of a journalistic nature (along with all the secretarial work and book-keeping, etc.). During the years 1967 to 1971 I was a "patient" in psychoanalysis with a woman, Vera Pettit. She was a great help to me in that she gave me her personal support and gentle loving concern during the most difficult part of my life. Psychoanalysis could not help me to understand my life more clearly. This happened to me after I returned to Canada in 1972 and became involved in the women's movement. I am a member of the Vancouver Mental Patients' Association. I see my life being spent in the pursuit of personal and political change.

DOROTHY SMITH was born in England in 1926. She completed her bachelor's degree in social anthropology at the London School of Economics in 1955, and a Ph.D. in sociology (two children later) at the University of California at Berkeley in 1963. She has published in the field of mental illness (her thesis was the study of the power structure of a state mental hospital), and on women in society. She is active in the women's movement and teaches women's studies and the sociology of knowledge at the University of British Columbia.

Press Gang is a small feminist printing and publishing collective. We do all the editing, layout and printing of all our titles. We are committed to the development of the print medium as a way of further understanding the political implications of our role as women/workers in a capitalist society. As a publisher, we want to make available a wide variety of literature that critically examines the role of women in Canada, countering the confining sexual stereotypes which oppress us and our children.

We also print for other organizations and individuals. As printers we reserve the right to control the end to which our skills and equipment are used. We refuse to print anything that is racist, sexist or that supports the inequalities of capitalism.

Also available from Press Gang

WOMEN'S WORK – a pamphlet by the Working Women's Assn.

FISHMARKET AND OTHER POEMS by Phyllis Baker

THE ANTI-PSYCHIATRY BIBLIOGRAPHY – researched and written by K. Portland Frank, Mental Patients Assn. 2nd edition, expanded and revised

JODY SAID – a collection of poetry by Beth Jankola

MUKTU, The Backward Muskox – a children's book by Heather Kellerhals-Stewart, illustrated by Karen Muntean